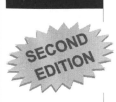

SECOND EDITION

42 Rules™ to Fight Dog Cancer (2ⁿᵈ Edition)

Real Stories and Practical Approaches to Dealing with Dog Cancer

By Aimee Quemuel
Foreword by Laurie Kaplan

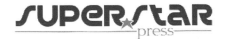

ſUPERſtAR press

E-mail: info@superstarpress.com
20660 Stevens Creek Blvd., Suite 210
Cupertino, CA 95014

Published by Super Star Press™, a Happy About® imprint 20660 Stevens Creek Blvd., Suite 210, Cupertino, CA 95014
http://42rules.com

2nd Edition: November 2012
1st Edition: August 2010
Paperback ISBN (2nd Edition): 978-1-60773-106-1 (1-60773-106-1)
Paperback ISBN (1st Edition): 978-1-60773-030-9 (1-60773-030-8)
eBook ISBN: 978-1-60773-031-6 (1-60773-031-6)
Place of Publication: Silicon Valley, California, USA
Library of Congress Number: 2010923749

Trademarks

Warning and Disclaimer

Praise For This Book!

"Having access to information such as what Aimee shares in her book has been reassuring and so educational. She has made this journey of fighting dog cancer a little more bearable, and inspired hope and optimism."
Annick Fournier, Owner of Anouch, Golden Retriever with Cancer

"42 Rules to Fight Dog Cancer is all about the HERO's journey we are invited to walk when our dog has been given a cancer diagnosis. This journey often feels like a 'fight.' As you will discover the 'Rules' are really about learning to navigate this journey in a way that honors ourselves, our dog and the special bond we share. This is the true essence of healing. This is the gift we are invited to receive."
Liz Fernandez, DVM, Acupuncture for Pets

"After reading 42 Rules to Fight Dog Cancer, I am impressed with the concise approach the book offers on not only DEALING with a dog who has cancer, but also methods and steps on how to AVOID the possibility of contracting a cancerous disease. When we are faced with a tough challenge in our dog's life, it's comforting to know that this book will give you the direction and guidance to get you through your challenge. A MUST READ for any dog owner."
Mark Siebel, Owner - Lead Trainer/Behaviorist at DOGGIE STEPS Dog Training, LLC.

"42 Rules to Fight Dog Cancer is a great guide full of helpful tips. It is a must read for anyone facing the dreaded diagnosis of cancer for his or her pet. Following the information in this book will give your pet the best chance of fighting this horrible disease."
Shawn Messonnier, DVM and award-winning author of *The Natural Vet's Guide to Preventing and Treating Cancer in Dogs*

Dedication

This book is dedicated to my beloved Cody and to all the dogs and their owners who are currently fighting or have fought dog cancer. You are forever in my heart.

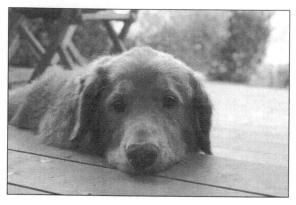

Cody Boy: November 8, 1995–April 7, 2008
Survived cancer 519 days

Acknowledgments

There are so many people to thank for this book. First, I'd like to thank the contributors to this book, as without them, there would be nothing to be thankful for. I would also like to say thank you to my incredible friends and family, who provided me with continuous support and encouragement during and after Cody's cancer ordeal.

I especially would like to say thanks to those who went above and beyond the call of duty towards the end of Cody's life when he became paralyzed. This was an extremely stressful time for me, as it challenged me not only emotionally but also physically, as I had to move around a 75-pound dog. To Chelsea and David Linn, who helped me clean the feces off Cody when he first went down while we were in San Francisco. To my brother, Geoffrey Quemuel, who made Cody a special sling to help keep the circulation going in his legs. To my dad, Nestor Quemuel, who not only allowed Cody to swim in his pool, but also helped me in the grueling task of getting him in and out of his life jacket, which, without back legs, was not easy. To my mom, Joscelyn Quemuel, who would bring me food to keep my strength going. To my sister, Jinky Mosdale, for graciously putting up with a very sick dog in our then shared home. To my very dear friends, especially Aura Gonzales-Kuehl, who provided me with much needed emotional support despite the death of her father.

You are the people that touched my heart in ways I cannot explain and I will never forget.

Contents

Foreword by Laurie Kaplan

In July 2000, I found out that my dog had cancer. I was shocked and devastated. Bullet was a strong, healthy, nine-year-old Siberian Husky and it was hard for me to believe that he had cancer. Thanks to my background as a researcher and medical animal writer, I was able to quickly gather the information I needed to formulate an attack plan. It was an all-out war, and I'm happy to say that we beat Bullet's cancer.

No matter how much information you accumulate, there is just no substitute for the sharing of stories. In this book, Aimee Quemuel has compiled wonderful canine cancer stories from people who fought (or are fighting) cancer for their dogs. Some are survival stories, some are not, but all will give you vital information and support in addition to some of the most heart-warming outpourings of love you will find anywhere. Each story illuminates one of Aimee's forty-two rules to fight dog cancer. The stories bring each rule to life by providing personal, real-life experiences in support of that rule. The rules that Aimee chose to include do a great job of covering some of the most important things to do and not to do if your dog has cancer.

A few of the stories you'll read were submitted by people who put their dogs through cancer treatment with help from the Magic Bullet Fund (MBF). As you might have guessed from the name, I founded this fund in honor of my boy Bullet. MBF provides financial assistance for people who have a dog with cancer, but cannot afford treatment costs. To date, the fund has seen eighty-six beautiful dogs through treatment that would not have had treatment without our help. The fund subsists on donations from individuals and corporations. You can apply for help or make a donation at http://www.themagicbulletfund.org.

The sharing of stories is an ancient art. In *42 Rules to Fight Dog Cancer*, Aimee provides a valuable resource of canine cancer rules and stories, but she doesn't stop there. Aimee also created an oasis on the Internet where we can share and pass on to new generations of dog lovers information that will help them, educate them, and encourage them to fight dog cancer.

Aimee's web site keeps the art of storytelling alive to help people who have dogs with cancer. At http://www.fightdogcancer.com, you'll see many stories by people fighting canine cancer. Read them to share the writer's discoveries, experiences, thoughts, and feelings. Some stories will show you what others have done for their dogs with the same type of cancer that you're fighting, and whether it worked or not. You'll find ideas that will help you make treatment decisions, diet decisions, and choices of supplements or alternative treatments. And, while you're there, don't forget to share your story with people who will truly understand and value your commitment, determination, and emotional investment.

Thank you, Aimee, for writing and compiling *42 Rules*. The advice you offer is invaluable, and anyone who has a dog with cancer will benefit from reading these moving stories by others who have had to fight for their dogs' lives.

Laurie Kaplan
Author, *Help Your Dog Fight Cancer*,
http://www.HelpYourdogFightCancer.com
Founder, Magic Bullet Fund,
http://www.TheMagicBulletFund.org

When my Golden Retriever, Cody, was diagnosed with hemangiosarcoma, an incurable blood cancer, I was devastated. He was the one who had been there through some of most transformative years of my life—from a bright-eyed college student to a hopefully still bright-eyed, but wiser, mid-thirty-year-old woman. The thought of losing him was unbearable.

Like most, I hit the Internet to try to make sense of it all. What I found was so disheartening: statistic after statistic predicting the demise of my boy. When I tried to find survival stories to draw inspiration from, they were far and few in between to say the least. It took me countless weeks and late-night hours to gather the information I needed to put together a treatment plan—all while trying to keep strong for my boy.

Experts predict that half of all dogs will get some type of cancer in their lifetimes with 80 percent of dogs over the age of ten dying from the disease. The statistics go on and on. But the good news is that for every dog that is diagnosed with cancer, there are thousands of stories of survival yet to be told. That is how the idea of *42 Rules to Fight Dog Cancer* came into existence.

42 Rules to Fight Dog Cancer is a compilation of real stories, told by real people about their dog cancer battles—21 different contributors in all. The book does not discriminate on type of treatment used, but all authors do have one thing in common: their dogs survived significantly longer than their prognoses. Some of the dogs in this book went into complete remission; some eventually succumbed to the cancer. Collectively, the dogs in this book survived 633 months with cancer, which means we got to spend that much more time with our pups. Take, for example, the amazing Disnay (pronounced Disney), a New Jersey Beagle owned by Robin Barbosa. Disnay not only beat the cancer odds and lived six and a half years after her diagnosis, but lived longer than most non-cancer dogs to the ripe old age of sixteen. The stories of survival are out there; you just need to dig a little to find them.

On a related note, I had several veterinarians and experts offer to provide their recommended treatment plans for the book, but that is not what this book is about. There are other books that provide more complete dog cancer treatment information like Laurie Kaplan's *Help Your Dog Fight Cancer*, or *The Natural Vet's Guide to Preventing and Treating Cancer in Dogs* and *Unexpected Miracles: Hope and Holistic Healing for Pets*, by Shawn Messonnier, DVM.

While there are lots of concrete tips that you can start using immediately in this book, it is not meant to be an exhaustive guideline on dog cancer treatments nor is it meant to replace the advice of your veterinarian. Rather, it is intended to provide a blend of inspirational stories and tips you can use right away in your dog cancer fight. Some authors give tips on specific treatments, others on the art of battling dog cancer. In the end, these are the recommended lessons learned from real owners who have fought or are fighting dog cancer.

An important note: **100 percent** of the author's proceeds will be donated to dog cancer nonprofits. By buying this book, you are joining us in our fight against dog cancer. We truly believe that together, with our collective knowledge, we can save our dogs.

1 Rules Are Meant to Be Broken

Aimee Quemuel

> Could you imagine if no one ever broke a rule? Progress would stop altogether. But if you broke the rules every time, mayhem would ensue. Rules have to change and evolve over time, or we simply don't grow.

"Cancer is a word, not a sentence." I first heard those words in the Sumner Foundation support group for dogs with hemangiosarcoma. They have stuck with me since that very first day Cody was diagnosed.

Those words embrace the spirit of our fight against dog cancer: *rules are meant to be broken*. Could you imagine if no one ever broke a rule? Progress would stop altogether. But if you broke the rules every time, mayhem would ensue. Rules have to change and evolve over time, or we simply don't grow.

If you are like most dog owners who are battling or who have battled dog cancer, you likely received a grim prognosis. Let the contributors of this book be proof that you have to take the "rules" of prognosis with a grain of salt. It is just a guess. No one—not even your veterinarian—knows for sure how *your* dog will respond to treatment.

There are thousands of dogs who have outlived their "sentence" and the twenty-one contributors to this book are prime examples that rules can be broken, especially when it comes to the statistical aspects of dog cancer. Each of them have beat their dog cancer prognosis and lived with cancer for more than a year and, in several cases, several years. Collectively, the book's authors enjoyed 633 more months with their dogs.

In Cody's battle, I was told to euthanize him on the spot, as he would surely not live more than a few days. But as discussed in Rule 4, Don't Make Rash Decisions to Euthanize, Sherri Cooper and I cover why, in some cases, listening to your heart—not just the voice of scientific reason—is the prudent path. Luckily, I listened to my heart, and Cody lived 519 more days.

In Rule 15, Do Something, Eric Johnson talks about how he stopped the pain medications and put his dog Kita on an herbal regimen, resulting in 17 more months.

On the flip side, there are some rules that never should be broken, like in the case of Karen Summers and her dog Tensing, whose initial "unconventional" chemotherapy protocol recommended by his regular veterinarian kicked Tensing out of remission. In particular, when it comes to dosage and administration of conventional therapies such as radiation, chemotherapy, steroids, and surgery, breaking the rules is a big no-no.

As the decision maker for your dog, you have the unfortunate and fortunate position to decide when to break the rules and when to follow them. It is a balancing act for sure, and only you can decide when to bend the rules and when you must hold steadfast. It is part instinct, part knowledge of your dog, and a whole lot of education.

Speaking on behalf of the 21 contributors of this book, we wish you knowledge, strength, and insight as you start this battle. We have all been in the same position you are in. We know how it feels. But we also know that whatever this journey brings you—whether you are lucky enough to get extra time with your dog or not—the fact that you are reading this book means you are doing something to fight, and that in itself is something to be proud of.

2 Never Stop Reading

Aimee Quemuel, Elizabeth Heller,
and Caryn Wilson

Remember that all action plans start with knowledge. So keep on reading. Keep on learning.

As the cliché goes, knowledge is power. When you first get the cancer diagnosis, no doubt you will hit the Internet and try to learn as much as possible about what lies ahead.

The more you know, the easier it is to make a decision. However, with so many resources available, and more and more informational sites popping up every day, it is hard to decide what information to trust. In addition, many cleverly disguised content sites are, in actuality, tied to a commercial product, so keep that in mind when reviewing such content.

I wish there was an easy answer to the credibility conundrum, but there isn't. But if you keep reading, you will start to see some continual themes. And that is your first clue to this process. In other words, if you start to see a treatment, approach, or suggested remedy over and over again, investigate it, as there is likely some kernel of truth to it.

Here are just a few examples of how knowledge can lead to action.

- One article I found revealed the possibilities of anti-angiogenesis protocols. From there, I found a local veterinarian that specialized in such protocols, specifically for Cody's cancer type. I believe this treatment, combined with the diet and supplements, gave him 519 extra days of life. It all started with reading and learning about my new dog cancer reality.

- Elizabeth Heller of Lexington, Massachusetts, read a book titled *Sharks Don't Get Cancer*,[i] which led her to a veterinarian in Texas who used a shark cartilage regimen for treating cancer. Elizabeth credits the treatment with three more quality years of life with her beloved Miniature Schnauzer Osquer. Again, it all started with reading.

- Caryn Wilson of Andover, Massachusetts, spent many nights researching and surfing the Web to help her decide on her Rottweiler Beanny's treatment plan. Beanny was six and a half when he was diagnosed with osteosarcoma and was given a year at most to live. During her research process, Caryn read of an herbal remedy called Essiac tea. Beanny lived twenty-one months post his diagnosis, and Caryn credits the Essiac tea. Once again, it started with reading.

If you are new to the dog cancer fight, putting together a research framework is also a helpful exercise. With a background in journalism, I reverted to one of the tried, true, and simple approaches to research: who, what, why, how, where, and when. Once I established this framework, almost every piece of research I found could be categorized and organized in a way that made sense to me. Here is an explanation of a research framework you could use. See Appendix B, for an example of what Cody's research map looked like and the correlating action plan.

Who: What is my dog's breed, and what diseases is the breed predisposed to?

What: What is the type of cancer and how does it work?

Why: What possibly caused my dog's cancer?

> **NOTE:** This is not about blame, but about learning. For example, research shows that lawn pesticides are a likely contributing cause of lymphoma. By knowing this, you can avoid its use as you move forward.

Where: Where are the tumors located?

When: How long does my veterinarian expect my dog to live?

How: How are others treating their dogs?

Remember that all action plans start with knowledge. I spent countless hours on the Internet. I set up a news feed so the latest dog cancer research was delivered to my desktop I read blogs and joined a support group. I read dozens of dog cancer books. The sum of my research translated into my treatment plan. So keep on reading. Keep on learning.

3 Gather a Team of Cancer-Fighting Experts

Ilene Powell

You have to go beyond your regular veterinarian and amass a group of experts to help guide you in your dog cancer fight.

Diagnosed at seven years old, Labrador Retriever Mali survived hemangiosarcoma more than four years through use of an integrative approach. Mali's owner, Ilene Powell, recommends that you gather an expert cancer-fighting team beyond just your regular veterinarian.

If you are like most, you likely received the initial cancer diagnosis from your regular veterinarian. However, cancer is a very specialized disease that requires specialized care. As such, you have to go beyond your regular veterinarian and amass a group of experts to help guide you in your dog cancer fight. Your team may include specialists in veterinary surgery, oncology, holistic care, pathology, imaging, nutrition, and/or other areas, depending on your individual needs.

So, why is this important? Your veterinarian is likely great at diagnosing, but as a generalist, he or she simply does not deal with dog cancer on a day-to-day basis. And if you do decide to do surgery or chemotherapy, wouldn't you rather work with a specialist vs. a generalist?

For example, veterinarian oncology is a specialized field of veterinary medicine. They have focused training on animals with cancer. Depending on your needs, the oncologist can oversee your dog's treatment, or he or she can assist your general practice veterinarian by sharing knowledge and techniques, or even participating as needed in surgeries and chemotherapy. An oncologist will be current on the best conventional treatments available, and will have firsthand experience treating hundreds of animals that have been diagnosed with cancer. Chemotherapy, immunotherapy, radiation therapy, and photodynamic therapy are each possible conventional treatments for your dog's cancer, and each method has pros and cons. A knowledgeable oncologist should be able to explain the details of each method.

When I decided on chemotherapy as part of Mali's regimen, I knew I had to consult with an oncologist. I was lucky in that my regular veterinarian flew in an oncologist for weekly treatments of his cancer patients. However, if there is not a local oncologist available in your area, an alternative is to have your regular veterinarian work with an oncologist remotely. There are several resources to help you find a remote oncologist such as Veterinary Oncology Consultants, http://www.vetoncologyconsults.com/.

Should you wish to add supplements such as vitamins and herbs, enhanced nutrition, and/or acupuncture to your dog's cancer arsenal, holistic veterinarians are well versed in these modalities. While I did not work with a holistic veterinarian, the oncologist we worked with had both Western and Eastern medical experience, so I had the added benefit of his expertise in this arena as well. He would regularly review my supplement list to ensure that they did not interfere with any of the conventional treatments we were using. While we wanted to do everything for her, everything may not have been right for Mali.

Once you gather the members of your team, try to build a personal relationship with them, with the goal of building a responsive, cancer-fighting team that rallies behind you. I brought my team food and sent them cards and pictures. I did the little things that made sure Mali and I were remembered. Keep in mind that your team is busy and you need to respect their time with other patients. Ask them how long it takes them to get back to you, and try to get their email addresses. Often, email is a better way for them to respond, especially after hours. And if you don't get a timely answer, keep following up, but again, be respectful.

4 Don't Make Rash Decisions to Euthanize

Aimee Quemuel and Sherri Cooper

Don't make the drastic, quick decision to put him down when you hear that scary word, "cancer." Give your dog a chance to fight the cancer.

The day after Cody collapsed at the beach due to a bleeding tumor caused by his cancer, I was literally seconds away from euthanizing him. Sleep deprived and extremely distraught, I sat in the veterinarian room with him for hours, hoping for a sign. That sign came in the form of something that Cody did everyday: begging for food. My friend Michael Kovacs was the one that actually saved his life. He playfully teased him with a jar of biscuits on the counter. Though a little on the weak side, Cody got up and barked like he always did when he wanted something.

That is when it hit me. The answer was so clear. He was not in obvious pain. Cody was still up for a biscuit, so he was still up for life. And, yes, while the prognosis was grim, it didn't mean that we had to let Cody go at the exact moment of time. In fact, Cody likely had cancer for months or even years before his actual diagnosis. I just didn't know it. So I never had to face the possibility of euthanasia.

With my decision made to wait it out, I brought Cody home for what I called his "last supper." I invited all who loved him to say their goodbyes. I cooked him a meal of meat and vegetables. I slept on the floor with him and prayed for a peaceful passing. Cody had 519 more "last suppers" and the decision *not to make a rash decision* made that possible.

Through the process of writing this book, I have heard of countless similar stories. Like Sherri Cooper and her English Mastiff Asia. When Asia was diagnosed with stomach cancer and given a grim prognosis, Sherri's whole world was turned upside down. One of her first thoughts was to euthanize. However, after the initial shock of the cancer diagnosis wore off, Sherri decided to at least try treatment. Twenty months later, as of this writing, Asia is living out her senior years in Okemos, Michigan, cancer-free.

"Don't make the drastic, quick decision to put him down when you hear that scary word, 'cancer.' Give your dog a chance to fight the cancer," advises Sherri.

Obviously, the decision to euthanize your dog is a very personal choice, and there is no right or wrong answer. Some say the decision to euthanize comes when the dog "can no longer live the life of a dog—and only the owner knows when that really is," or when the dog's "suffering exceeds their ability to take pleasure in life." In Rule 41, Know When to Let Go, Laurie Kaplan gives some guidance on this topic.

If Cody was in obvious pain, I would have certainly leaned towards letting him go. In fact, that is the decision I had to make on April 7, 2008, but not before he had 519 days of living.

Remember that cancer is a word, not a sentence, and just because your dog is diagnosed with cancer today, does not mean that he can't have many more tomorrows.

5 Seek Open-Minded Veterinarians

Aimee Quemuel

Especially if you are not given any treatment options, seek open-minded veterinarians who are willing to explore safe options that just might help get you more time with your beloved dog.

Especially if you are not given any treatment options, seek open-minded veterinarians who are willing to explore safe options that just might help get you more time with your beloved dog. After getting seven "second opinions," it was easy to spot the veterinarians with open minds. They tended to have had the most recent schooling and access to the latest cutting edge technologies to cure dog cancer. When I brought up a treatment I read about, they would say something like, "Well, I have not heard of that, but based on the ingredients, it wouldn't do any harm, so it should be safe to at least try."

On the flip side, the "closed-minded" veterinarians I consulted with did not offer treatment plans beyond tramadol, a narcotic for relieving pain. While I understand that all the statistics said that Cody's cancer was considered incurable, it started to become apparent that some veterinarians are so by the book, and would default to what they knew best: the grim statistics. I even recall asking one of them about new anti-angiogenesis protocols for fighting cancer; she had no idea what I was talking about, and then proceeded to talk about how the cancer was incurable.

Five out of the seven veterinarians I consulted with all recommended that I euthanize Cody as he wouldn't last more than a few weeks. One even recommended that I keep his IV/PIC line, as she was positive I would be returning to euthanize him in a few days.

However, two veterinarians encouraged me to at least try. While they both still warned me of the grim statistics, they both helped me put together a treatment plan that put Cody into remission and gave me 17 more months with him.

Dr. Cadile from San Mateo Veterinary Medical Specialists, http://www.vmsmedicine.com/doctors.htm, was still in the process of doing her oncology medical residency program when I came to her. Not only was she full of piss and vinegar, she also was involved in cutting-edge studies on anti-angiogenic therapy for curing hemangiosarcoma. Dr. Cadile, prescribed Cody a new anti-angiogenesis program. While Dr. Cadile warned that she did not think it would help, she said it would not hurt to try. I believe it helped two out of the three tumors go into remission—as they were eventually undetectable via ultrasound.

The other was Dr. Molly Rice, of Coastal Holistic, http://www.coastalholistic.com/doctors.html. I brought Cody to her within the first few weeks of his diagnosis and she immediately began acupuncture treatment. She also recommended a few Chinese herbs to help him in his cancer battle. Again, she warned me of the grim statistics, but she helped me do something. That something translated into a cancer miracle story.

This is not to say that veterinarians who go only "by the books" can't help you, in fact, when it came to Cody's surgery to remove his spleen, I went with a veterinarian that had been doing surgery for 20+ years "by the book," as this was a time that I felt this kind of experience was critical. I just think that adding a few open-minded veterinarians will help round out your team. They provide a fresh perspective and are often the ones that have recently been in school, so they have been exposed to experiential treatment plans that might not have been passed on to "by the book" veterinarians yet.

6 Get a Second Opinion

Aimee Quemuel

If your veterinarian recommends a specific action plan, get a second opinion and ask other dog owners about their treatment plans.

Just days before Cody collapsed at the beach in San Francisco and was subsequently diagnosed with cancer, I went to my regular veterinarian as I knew something was wrong. His energy seemed low and he would hack during our regular walks. The veterinarian said he had a simple cough and prescribed a cough medicine. Four days later, Cody collapsed at the beach and was diagnosed with hemangiosarcoma and given a day or two to live.

While I was not happy about the misdiagnosis, I do believe that everything happens for a reason. Ironically, the misdiagnosis was the catalyst that drove many of the decisions I made for Cody. I started to view veterinarians as educated team members of my dog cancer team, not the final decision makers. They were the medical experts, but I was the expert on Cody. I am the one that knew him the best.

Prior to the misdiagnosis, I never questioned my veterinarian. I simply followed his or her orders. They were, after all, the experts.

I believe that when one is under the stress of a cancer diagnosis, sometimes it seems easier just to let someone else decide what to do. But if I let someone else decide Cody's fate, he would never have lived to see his twelfth birthday. I realize that I was one of the lucky ones. But my story is proof that it is possible.

While most of the veterinarians pretty much gave the same grim statistics I read on the Internet, something told me not to give up. If you have that same inkling, go with it. I knew Cody was not ready to go, and I also knew that my primary veterinarian was wrong about his original diagnosis, so it was possible that the veterinarians were also wrong about the outcome.

Each of the seven veterinarians, whether conventional or holistic, offered up at least one bit of wisdom. Sometimes I really had to listen to glean that nugget of wisdom, but even the most pessimistic veterinarians offered up something. So I took all those nuggets of wisdom and came up with my own plan of action.

If your veterinarian recommends a specific action plan, get a second opinion and ask other dog owners about their treatment plans. I have heard of too many nightmare stories in which a dog owner simply followed orders only to later find out that there was a better way or that the cancer was misdiagnosed.

Just recently, a fellow dog owner contacted me because her dog had a tumor on her spleen and liver. Her veterinarian said it was lymphoma. When I asked her if her veterinarian did a biopsy, she said no. How the heck the veterinarian knew it was lymphoma is beyond me. The spleen has already been removed and disposed of and now the owner is at a loss for what to do.

In Rule 13, Dosage Is as Important as the Treatment, Karen Summers talks about her ordeal in which bad advice from her veterinarian led to her dog Tensing falling out of remission. Again, if she had received a second opinion before acting, Karen believes that Tensing would still be alive.

Let me be clear. I am not saying that veterinarians are always wrong or that you should not listen to their advice. In fact, they were very much critical to Cody's dog cancer fight. But just remember they are humans. They make mistakes and they are fallible. Get second opinions and take advantage of their expertise to help guide you through the process, not make the decisions for you.

7 Have a Goal for Each Appointment

Aimee Quemuel

Dealing with cancer is emotional, confusing, and overwhelming, so you need to make sure you stay on track by having a specific goal for each visit. Personally, I am a list person so I went to each appointment with a written list of very specific questions. Obviously, the goal of each visit will depend on where you are at with your cancer battle.

However, if you are just starting this journey, keep in mind that the first few appointments are critical as they are what help you decide your treatment plan. To that end, here is a list of initial questions to ask during the start of your dog cancer battle. Of course, if you have others, add them to the list. And if you are not a good note taker, record your appointment or bring someone with you.

1. *If it were your dog, what would you do?* At the end of the day, you will need to decide the final treatment plan, but putting your veterinarian in your shoes can incent even the most conservative veterinarian to offer you some small sliver of hope. Asking this question can change the tone of the conversation. I can recall one of the more conservative veterinarians responding to this question by recommending an herbal remedy, "Hoxley formula," to treat Cody's cancer. Prior to that, he had simply said there was nothing we could do.

2. *Have you heard of any clinical trials for my dog's cancer?* Practicing veterinarians typically only use accepted protocols to treat cancer. Similar to human clinical trials, it can take years to bring cutting-edge treatment to the market. In other words, you have to seek out such clinical trials.

3. *Do you know of any "alternative" remedies that might help in my dog's cancer fight?* If you are going to a conventional veterinarian, this question is a must. Remember, your regular veterinarian likely only learned the Western modality to medicine, so, like most, he or she will stick to what he or she knows best.

4. *What are the expected outcomes and statistics?* While you have to take statistics with a grain of salt, it is important to know what you are dealing with.

5. *What are the possible side effects of drugs or treatments you are recommending?* Virtually every synthetic drug and even some herbs have a side effect. As such, you need to know what to expect and how to possibly curb unfavorably reactions.

6. *How much experience have you had with dog cancer, and my dog's specific cancer?* If your regular veterinarian is the one that diagnosed your dog, chances are that they don't deal with dog cancer on a daily basis, and you will want to know this before deciding to work with him or her on your dog's treatment.

7. *Do you recommend any specialists that I can consult with?* Your veterinarian is likely great at diagnosing your dog's cancer, but is certainly not a specialist when it comes to dog cancer treatment. And if you do decide to do surgery or chemotherapy, wouldn't you rather work with a specialist vs. a generalist? Refer back to Rule 3, Gather a Team of Cancer-Fighting Experts.

8. *What are the potential costs?* Knowing how much treatment can cost is important so you can plan ahead. If you can't afford treatment, see Rule 11 by Rebecca Clark on innovative ways you can raise the funds needed for treatment. Don't give up hope just because of money.

Join a Support Group

Aimee Quemuel and Ilene Powell

Fighting canine cancer may not always be one-size-fits-all, and a fellow dog cancer story may be just the inspiration you need to try a treatment that may save your dog's life.

Battling dog cancer is an emotional roller coaster, for sure, and being surrounded by a community that understands exactly what you are going through is invaluable. There are dozens of support groups, all with a slightly different focus. Some are focused on specific cancer types, others are focused on dogs actively living with cancer and some are purely for support once your dog has passed. While members are typically not experts, they are fellow dog cancer fighters who can provide unique knowledge and experience that a veterinarian cannot offer; the kind of insight that can help you better prepare for the many decisions you will need to make on behalf of your dog. A partial list of support groups is provided in Appendix B.

Oftentimes, fellow dog owners can help prevent you from making the same mistake they did. For example, Karen Summers, contributor to this book, openly discusses how her dog fell out of remission due to a poorly implemented chemo protocol. This is the kind of information that you will not find anywhere else, but from some sort of support group. In a way, this book is like a support group experience. The members/ authors are not professionals, but they are witnesses and experts to their own dog cancer battles.

For dog owners sharing the information, it is often therapeutic. Plus, the people in support groups are real dog owners who have faced the same dog cancer ordeal. They usually don't have monetary interest in telling their story, which means the information they provide does not have any other motive but to help you have more time with your dog.

Veterinarians tend to be statistically driven, as this is how they are trained. They may give you some survival odds, which may be conservative for liability reasons and based on historical averages. But a dog owner, who has beaten the odds and shares his or her story, might provide you with a cutting edge treatment plan that you can at least investigate. Fighting canine cancer may not always be one-size-fits-all, and a fellow dog cancer story may be just the inspiration you need to try a treatment that may save your dog's life.

Dog owners need to believe that the "odds" can be just that…"odd." No one knows for sure your dog's ability to fight its cancer. Not even your veterinarian.

And last, but not least, joining a support group increases your chances of getting an immediate answer or at least some guidance on the question at hand. Sometimes that is enough to get you through the night. On several occasions, I can recall posting a question on a support group at 2:00 a.m., and within minutes someone responded. Dog owners fighting for their beloved pets' lives are dedicated and quite active, which means you will benefit from the sense of urgency that dog owners currently in battle will exhibit.

Ilene Powell sums it up best: "Reaching out is NOT a sign of weakness; it shows strength and control."

The Power of Positivity

Jeanne Arsenault

We all know the effects of positive energy and, despite the lack of scientific data to back it, even the most skeptical people turn to some sort of spiritual-based thinking in times of need.

At ten and a half years old, Jeanne Arsenault's Golden Retriever/Cocker Spaniel mix Bailey was diagnosed with prostate cancer and given three to four months to live with no treatment and ten months with chemo. Bailey survived twenty-one months after his initial diagnosis, with no conventional treatment, and died of natural causes. A completely natural approach that included healing sessions, a natural diet, and herbs was used in this success story. No chemo or surgery.

Just months after I lost my father to the dreaded disease, my beloved Bailey was diagnosed with prostate cancer. The doctors advised me that my Bailey had only three to four months to live, but with chemo we might be able to extend his life by six more months.

For months prior to his diagnosis, I saw my father battle this disease and watched helplessly as it took its effect on his body and spirit; a scenario I didn't want to see repeated with Bailey. As the voice for Bailey, I had the unfortunate and fortunate position of having to make all of his decisions. He couldn't verbally tell me what he wanted, but I knew my old dog would never survive chemo and, above all, I didn't want to see him suffer.

Since I am a strong believer in holistic remedies (unfortunately, my father did not share my beliefs), I went online and studied alternative remedies to cancer. In addition to changing his diet and adding herbs/supplements to his regiment, I began what I referred to as "healing sessions" with Bailey. We all know the effects of positive energy and, despite the lack of scientific data to back it, even the most skeptical people turn to some sort of spiritual-based thinking in times of need.

I would begin by putting on soft, meditative music. I would then place my hands on his body, particularly in the areas of his heart, lungs, and prostate. I would breathe deeply into my body, and then I would envision positive energy flowing from me to him. I would imagine the blood running freely through his veins, into his heart and lungs, and I would picture all the organs in his body functioning properly.

I would envision the tumor in his prostate shrinking until there was nothing of it left in his body. As I would perform this ritual, I would begin to feel the energy running down my arms, out of my fingertips and into his body, like a flow of electricity. As I would feel the sensation, I always knew when it would reach his body, as he would jolt just slightly and then he would lift his head and look directly at me. This happened each time, without exception. I would perform these sessions at least once a week, sometimes more often if he was feeling particularly low on energy. After these sessions, he would be more alert and lively, often acting like a young dog again.

I am convinced that his new diet and the healing sessions are the reason that twenty-one months after Bailey was given four months to live, he was diagnosed cancer-free and able to live his life to the ripe old age of nearly thirteen—the equivalent to roughly ninety-one human years.

Forget Your Beliefs in Modalities

Lynn Browne

Whether you believe in Western or Eastern modalities, when it comes down to it, the goal is more quality time with your dog.

At thirteen years old, Samson, a Great Pyrenees, was diagnosed with incurable hemangiosarcoma of the spleen and given three months to live, even with surgery. Using a combination of Western and Eastern approaches, Samson is living out his senior years in Greenfield Center, New York, with his owner Lynn Browne. At the time of this writing, Sampson has survived seventeen cancer-free months.

Weighing in at eighty pounds, Samson has always been small for his breed. But what he lacks in size, he makes up for in heart and persistence. My former dog Alex cleverly tried to lose him twice when he was a puppy. But Samson just kept coming back. Nothing, even a dog purposely trying to lose him, was going to keep Samson from his home.

Never sick a day, Samson had thirteen very healthy years, but I knew something was wrong in June 2008 when my sweet boy barely had the energy to lift his head. His gums were white and he stopped eating all together. He wouldn't even lick an ice cube.

Accustomed to a healthy Samson, I was thoroughly shocked when he was diagnosed with incurable hemangiosarcoma of the spleen. It seemed so strange that one day I had a seemingly healthy dog, and the next day, one in dire health. It just didn't seem right.

Hemangiosarcoma, as it turns out, causes bleeding tumors. It is probably one of the worst cancers in dogs in terms of cure rates. Statistically speaking, it is considered incurable. Dogs with this cancer usually bleed to death due to erupting tumors. Samson was rushed to the veterinarian for emergency surgery to remove his spleen, which would stop the massive bleeding. Luckily, the tumor had not spread, but the bleed out meant that the cancer cells were released into his blood stream.

With a background in alternative healing, I have always felt that a blending of the two worlds—Eastern and Western—was ideal when dealing with any health issue. With the help of Western medicine in the form of surgery by my primary veterinarian, Samson was given a second chance. But I knew that I had to address the underlying cause of the cancer. I had to get his system back in balance. And that is where Eastern medicine came in.

Often referred to as "alternative medicine" by the Western world, Eastern medicine has been practiced for thousands of years and is actually older than the Western approach, which has only been around for the past hundred years.

Determined to get Samson's system back in balance so his body could fight the cancer in the first place, I embarked on the second part of Samson's cancer battle. I found a veterinarian specializing in Chinese medicine, who made him a custom blend of Chinese herbs. In addition, Samson now gets regular chiropractic adjustments, and I have also changed his diet accordingly. Lastly, I make sure that both my primary and holistic veterinarians are in continual communication to ensure that all treatments both Western and Eastern—are working synergistically.

My biggest piece of advice for dog owners fighting dog cancer is to keep an open mind. By nature and via my background, I lean towards Eastern medicine. In that same token, I know of many people that lean towards the Western approach. Whether you believe in Western or Eastern modalities, when it comes down to it, the goal is more quality time with your dog. So take the best from both worlds. That is what I did and the results speak for themselves. My boy Samson, the dog who was only given a few months to live, has been cancer-free for seventeen months.

11 Funding Your Cancer Fight

Rebecca Clark

People—even strangers—love animals and are willing to help you, but you have to seek out assistance.

Canine cancer treatment requires a substantial financial outlay, ranging between $600 and $6,000 per dog. Many dog owners cannot support such a large, unanticipated expense. And, in the case of Rebecca Clark from Newport, Rhode Island, who was suddenly faced with two dogs with cancer, the expenses were just too much.

I have heard of dog owners who tragically have had to euthanize their dogs because they just did not have the money to pay for treatment, or they weren't aware of the options out there for treatment. Kibo is living proof that this does not have to happen. People—even strangers—love animals and are willing to help you, but you have to seek out assistance.

My life was first affected by canine cancer in 2006, when my Yellow Lab, Sana, age six at the time, was diagnosed with mast cell cancer. He had three surgeries to remove the tumors and the veterinarian was able to get clean margins, which gave him a good prognosis. It was not easy, but I paid for Sana's surgery and treatment out of my own pocket.

Then, in December 2008, cancer reared its ugly head once again when my other Yellow Lab, Kibo, was diagnosed with lymphoma at age eleven. I was not only heartbroken, but worried about how I would pay for his expensive chemo treatments. That is when I learned of the Magic Bullet Fund, http://www.themagicbulletfund.org.

The Magic Bullet Fund (MBF) provides financial assistance for canine cancer treatment when the family is financially unable to provide treatment. Most families contribute some portion of the treatment fees, and MBF contributes only the amount that the family cannot pay. In addition, there are other organizations such as the Dog and Cat Cancer Fund™, http://www.dccfund.org, and the Canine Cancer Awareness group, http://caninecancerawareness.org, that help dog owners fund their dog cancer fights.

I immediately applied to the MBF and thankfully was accepted, as I would not have been able to begin Kibo's cancer treatment without their help and, with cancer, time is of the essence. In addition, my friend created a Web site for Kibo where people could go online and contribute. I sent that along with the MBF information to anyone I could think of. I even posted in the pet section of Craigslist and received some donations in that manner.

Then something amazing happened. One of our local newspapers heard about Kibo through a Magic Bullet Fund press release and did a story on him. I was *shocked* when my veterinarian called a few days later and said more than $2,000 had been sent in to help with Kibo's veterinarian bills. I literally sobbed in relief, and hope. One couple, whom I had never met, sent in $1700 in memory of their Yellow Labs, MacGyver and Max, both of whom were lost to cancer. The staff at a local donut place I had never been to collected $500 amongst them. A man from another part of the state, again someone I didn't know, sent $400. A small local business sent $5, and many other people sent varying amounts to help Kibo. It was one of the most beautiful gestures from humanity that I have ever experienced and it gave me hope and strength to fight for and with Kibo.

Thanks to the generosity of my friends, family, and dog lovers around the world, Kibo lived 412 day post his diagnosis. I am eternally grateful for every extra day my daughter and I had with our boy. Very sadly, we lost Sana in June of 2009 due to a mast cell cancer recurrence.

Though we lost Kibo to cancer, I am glad that money, or the lack thereof, was not the deciding factor in his fate. And, of course, I am forever grateful to those who have enabled Kibo to fight this vicious disease.

Tailor Your Dog's Treatment Plan

Aimee Quemuel

Find out exactly how your dog's cancer "acts out" and fight it with tools aimed squarely at supporting that specific organ or proven techniques for getting your dog into remission.

While there are some steps you can take with any cancer—like changing the diet, stopping vaccinations, boosting the immune system, and removing carcinogens from your dog's environment—every cancer is slightly different. As such, I highly recommend that you tailor your dog's treatment to combat the specifics of his or her cancer. Find out exactly how your dog's cancer "acts out" and fight it with tools aimed squarely at supporting that specific organ or proven techniques for getting your dog into remission.

Cody was originally diagnosed because he collapsed due to a bleed out in his heart. They had to drain fluid and blood from his heart and informed me that he would surely bleed out again and I would need to either drain his heart again or let him go. His heart never bled out again. And I believe it was because of something called Yunnan Paiyao.

I found out from a fellow dog owner fighting hemangiosarcoma that a Chinese herb called Yunnan Paiyao is said to stop massive internal and external bleeding and is highly recommended for any dog with hemagiosarcoma. In fact, further research revealed that the Viet Cong used Yunnan Paiyao to stop massive bleeding in the Vietnam War. They would pour the powder directly on gunshot wounds and would also take it internally to stop bleeding. I figured that Cody was given only a few days to live, so I might as well try it. So within the first day of Cody's diagnosis, he was on Yunnan Paiyao to help curb any massive bleeding events. This would also buy me time so that all the supplements and herbal remedies would have the necessary time to heal his body. As a side note, I later cut my hand while cooking and tested it out for myself. And guess what? The bleeding stopped immediately. It is now a staple ingredient in my first aid kit.

The only reason I used this herb was because I knew how his cancer worked. He had a blood-born cancer called hemangiosarcoma with tumors in his heart, spleen, and liver. Hemangiosarcoma causes bleeding tumors. Dogs with this cancer typically pass from bleeding to death. Chemo is not typically effective for this cancer, especially once metastasized. On the other hand, based on what I have learned in the past few years, if he had lymphoma, I would have seriously considered chemotherapy since there is an 80–90 percent success rate with this particular cancer.

In addition, I put Cody on supplements to fight tumors on his specific organs. For his liver, I used the herbal remedy milk thistle. According to Wikipedia, milk thistle (silymarin), sometimes called Mary thistle and holy thistle, is a flowering herb related to the daisy and ragweed family and is a well-known natural treatment for liver problems. It is also very safe to use.

For his heart, I included the supplement Coenzyme Q10 (CoQ10) and the herbal remedy hawthorn berry—both touted as natural heart support and, again, both safe at the recommended doses. According to the web site WebMD, CoQ10 is present throughout the body and, according to some clinical studies, supplementation with CoQ10 is a beneficial treatment of patients with congestive heart failure. Hawthorn berry is made from the tiny red berries as well as the leaves and flowers that grow on the hawthorn shrub (Crataegus oxyacantha). The herbal extract has been used in traditional medical systems since ancient times and is widely used as a heart tonic, particularly in Europe.[ii]

Cody also received weekly acupuncture with special emphasis on supporting his affected organs.

If I had to do it all over again, I would have added additional herbal support for Cody's spleen. Ironically, that is the only tumor that did not go away naturally. The tumors in his heart (equaling 2x5 centimeters) and liver (several nodules) were undetectable via ultrasound after five months of nutrition and herbal therapy. The veterinarians were amazed and said they had never seen this. Cody's cancer was considered incurable and regression of tumors without surgery is typically unheard of.

13 Dosage Is as Important as Treatment

Karen Summers

Whether you use chemotherapy, radiation, or some other conventional or natural treatment, dosage and administration are just as important as the treatment itself.

This next rule comes from Karen Summers of Sparta, Missouri, whose Siberian Husky, Tensing, was diagnosed with lymphoma and lived two years past the original diagnosis.

After my dog's cancer was discovered, I learned that dogs with lymphoma have excellent survival rates when treated with chemotherapy—80 to 90 percent—so there was no question that we would use chemo for Tensing. In addition, the quality of life is excellent for dogs on chemo and, in most cases, the dogs don't even get sick, and they don't usually lose their hair. During the entire chemo treatment Tensing only got sick twice.

However, despite the excellent survival rates, what I didn't know at the time was just how critical administration and dosage are to successful treatment. Unfortunately, I learned the hard way that the administration of the chemo protocol is just as important as the chemo itself.

After ten treatments, my original veterinarian told me that Tensing was in remission and we could now stop treatment. But quickly after chemo stopped, Tensing fell out of remission. I was confused as to how Tensing could fall out of remission so quickly.

So I started to do more research, which resulted in my questioning my original veterinarian's chemo protocol. I also discovered other supportive therapies, such as a low carbohydrate diet to ensure that I was not feeding the cancer. In addition, I discovered the importance of removing any environmental toxins from Tensing's environment, such as harsh chemicals commonly used in a home.

In my research, I came across Laurie Kaplan, founder of the Magic Bullet Fund (MBF), an organization that raises funds for dog owners that can't afford their dogs' cancer treatments, and author of *Help Your Dog Fight Cancer*, a tribute to Laurie's dog, Bullet, that also includes a crash course on how to care for dogs with cancer. Just like Tensing, Bullet was a Siberian Husky who had lymphoma. Bullet lived four-plus years past his original diagnosis and died cancer-free. I wanted the same for my Tensing.

Reaching out to Laurie was one of the best things I could have done. It was the turning point that helped Tensing get on a chemo protocol administered in the most effective manner. In talking with Laurie, I quickly found out that when a chemo protocol is stopped midstream, remission is also very likely to end.

The way the chemo was originally administered to Tensing was questionable at best. Tensing was kept overnight during every chemo treatment, as he was being given 18-hour infusions and was left unattended in a clinic cage. This breaks the first law in infusion therapy, not to mention the isolation and stress to my dog. I later found out that treatments should take anywhere from twenty minutes to two hours at most, and it is very risky to abandon a protocol midstream—neither of which were followed by my original veterinarian.

The bottom line is whether you use chemotherapy, radiation, or some other conventional or natural treatment, dosage and administration are just as important as the treatment itself.

When using chemo, for example, typically protocols should not be stopped midstream, especially when you are ahead of the cancer and the dog is feeling excellent. Chemo protocols are usually sixteen weeks, and once you decide on chemo as your course of action, you have to see it through—unless, of course, the dog is too sick for treatment or not responding to or tolerating the treatment. Tensing lived two more years past his diagnosis, which I am eternally grateful for. But I do believe that if the chemo had been done correctly, my beautiful Tensing would be here today and looking forward to another snowy winter.

Fight for Your Dog

Suzanne Morrone

Don't be afraid to stand up and fight for your dog. Make sure everyone understands that your dog is family.

Contrary to the stereotype of her breed, Zara, a Pit Bull/Wolf Mix, was a gentle, shy giant and mother figure to the all the animals in the house. At seven years old she was diagnosed with mast cell cancer and given a poor prognosis without further treatment. Surgery, aggressive radiation that required four to five hours of daily driving, and lots of love were the treatments that her owner Suzanne Morrone decided upon, giving Zara another six years of quality life.

Once you decide on a treatment plan, my advice is this: don't be afraid to stand up and fight for your dog. Make sure everyone understands that your dog is family. I told everyone—my friends, my work, the judge when I was picked for jury duty, and my husband—Zara comes first. I never regretted my choice for one second. We fought hard and were rewarded with six more years.

With a dominant dog named Hopi already in our home, I knew that adding to our pack would be challenging. However, from the very beginning, Zara was meant to grace my life. I happened to stop at my neighbor's house to "just see" his puppies when, out of nowhere, this little puppy shot across the yard and into my arms.

From that day forward, and despite a shy demeanor with strangers, Zara not only became my girl, but also the mother figure both to our many animals and to our small grandchildren. Hopi, the once dominant, feral dog we rescued from the Hopi Reservation in Arizona, took to

Zara immediately. She was his dog. So much so that Zara even became his seizure alert. Prior to a seizure, she would run between him and me barking until I made sure he was safe. This happened time and time again. It was absolutely amazing. And when my cat had kittens, she watched their birth, and protected them too. Even when a turtle got loose, Zara once again went into action, barking and racing to me until the turtle was safely back in its enclosure.

Zara had terrible allergies, so we had to bathe her frequently. Ironically, her allergies were both a curse and a blessing. Early in 1999, during one of her weekly baths, I found a tumor on the back of her hind leg. I immediately had the tumor removed and biopsied. Mast cell cancer was the diagnosis and, because of the location, the surgeon was not able to get clean margins. Without the further recommended radiation, Zara's prognosis was not good. I was given two options: radiation once a week in which Zara would be dropped off at a local veterinarian, crated, and then driven to Santa Cruz for treatment; or an exhaustive daily radiation treatment two hours away at UC Davis, a world-renowned veterinarian school. The latter choice not only offered a more aggressive protocol, but would also allow me to be by Zara's side. I wouldn't leave her to face this alone. So Zara, Hopi (my other dog and Zara's best friend), and I started on a month-long journey of daily radiation treatments, with weekly then monthly and bimonthly follow-up treatments for a full year. I literally had to stop my life so that my girl could have hers.

In the end, the mast cell cancer never came back, but she did get bone cancer at the site of radiation and we had to euthanize her. Zara, our angel of mercy, will live in my heart forever.

Do Something

Erik Johnson

Your emotional investment can prevent you from seeing beyond what your veterinarian tells you, and often you can fall into the trap of doing nothing but waiting for the inevitable.

At nine years old, Kita, Erik Johnson's Akita mix, was diagnosed with prostate and bladder cancer. Erik was told there was nothing he could do. But to Erik, doing nothing was simply unacceptable. So he decided to do something, and his tip is just that: try something, anything, just don't do nothing. Doing something in Erik's case bought his dog Kita seventeen more months of quality life, though his veterinarian gave him two months at most.

When Kita was first diagnosed, I felt desperate. Our only options were to administer pain pills or euthanize him on the spot. We decided to take him home and make him comfortable, the equivalent of hospice care for humans.

At first, we followed the veterinarian's orders and loaded Kita up on painkillers. But they just seemed to make him sick. He would vomit several times a day and it seemed to be linked to the pain medications that were supposed to make him feel better. For a dog that was so vibrant and full of life just months prior, it killed me to see him this way.

When scared, I think some people just freeze and stop thinking on their own. Your emotional investment can prevent you from seeing beyond what your veterinarian tells you, and often you can fall into the trap of doing nothing but waiting for the inevitable. That is what happened to me.

But luckily, we decided to take Kita off the pain medications to see what would happen, and, strangely, he was immediately better. This sudden reprieve from illness got me thinking. The veterinarian told me the pain pills would make him feel better, but they didn't. The veterinarian also said there was nothing we could do, but now I questioned that. Doing nothing just felt like giving up. And I was not about to give up on my loyal dog who would go everywhere with me.

I am in the herbal industry and eventually it dawned on me that I should try one of our products for my dog. Like I said, at first I was scared and thought I was doing the best I could for Kita if I just listened to the doctor's orders. But I believe in herbs and have seen first-hand the positive effects they can have on a person's health. What did I have to lose? After all, the veterinarian did not give me any options. So I opted to give it a shot. We put him on Uro Solution (canine) and Prostate Helper (for men) available at http://www.pet-helper.com and http://www.hls-herbs.com, respectively.

Within ten days, Kita was back to looking like a puppy again. His eyes got their color back and it was like the nightmare never happened.

For the next sixteen months, we went on several walks a day, and Kita was treated like every day could be his last. He was given all kinds of foods we normally would not have given him and a huge helping of love. This along with the herbal products really seemed to keep him in good health for a wonderful seventeen months in total from the time we got the original diagnosis.

All seemed to be going well, and it felt like Kita would go on forever. But then one day it was like a switch got turned and he lost the use of his legs. The veterinarians suspected that the cancer metastasized to his spine, interfering with neural activity. So, on Christmas Eve, we had to let him go.

I think that no matter how it happens, it is always difficult to lose your dog. However, as painful as it was to lose Kita, I think it would have been more painful if I had done nothing. This way, I know I gave him my best shot—he deserved that.

16

Let Your Dog Live Life to the Fullest

Lisa Alford and Pam Storto

Cancer, if you let it, can be that constant reminder that the days with your beloved dog are quickly slipping away.

There is no doubt that a cancer diagnosis is scary. But it does not mean life has to stop all together. If your dog is still with you, you still have time to enjoy life together. This next rule comes from Lisa Alford and Pam Storto, whose dogs were diagnosed at very young ages (just five and a half, and three and a half, respectively).

When Lucy, my beautiful white Great Dane, was hit with two different types of cancers (subcutaneous hemangiosarcoma and thyroid) plus heart disease (cardiomyopathy), I was heartbroken. Talk about a triple whammy, which was soon followed by emergency surgery for bloat. But I decided early on that I was not going to let the cancer diagnosis spoil my time with Lucy.

I know it is easier said than done, but you have to forget the prognosis—that's a human hang-up and simply an educated guess. Lucy was only given three months to a year to live if her heart didn't fail first. As of this writing in November 2009, she is still with me, nineteen months after her diagnosis. I realize that not everyone will be given this much extra time, but like the many authors of this book can attest to, it is possible. But you have to believe it in your heart, or it never will be. That is where it all starts.

Every living creature has a limited time on this earth. Intellectually, we all know this. But emotionally, now that is a different story. We dread the thought of death. Cancer, if you let it, can be that constant reminder that the days with your beloved dog are quickly slipping away. This is natural, of course. It is a constant mind battle for sure, but one that can be won.

I had to train myself to think differently. I told myself daily that Lucy had cancer way before the actual diagnosis and that during the "ignorant bliss" period I let her play and live life to the fullest. The only difference now is that I know she has cancer. But if you think about it, this is a good thing because with this knowledge, I can find ways to help prolong her life and, more importantly, maintain the quality of her life.

Pamela Storto, whose Golden Retriever, Sierra, battled lymphoma, advises, "You have to live each and every day to the fullest. Never look for tomorrow because you will miss what you have that day."

Pamela's dog Sierra was only three and half years old when she was diagnosed, and, despite her loss, she still reflects on the extra time as "thirteen wonderful additional months of life."

Some caveats: While I highly recommend you let your dog live life to the fullest, you will likely need to make some adjustments based upon your dog's cancer. In Lucy's case, we have to minimize sun exposure, as all white and light-colored dogs should, and prolonged activity. Lucy has always been a calm couch potato, but her favorite activity is enjoying the love and attention of people at events for Great Dane rescue. Since she now tires more easily, which limits her time at events, I had to get creative and find more opportunities for her to visit with people without putting her health at risk. So, in September 2009, after chemotherapy, surgery, and nutrition therapy, Lucy became an official therapy dog, visiting the pediatric floors at our local hospital. She absolutely loves it, and the smiles on the kids' faces when this beautiful, white dog with huge blues eyes walks into their rooms is a memory that I will keep forever. And you know what? Sometimes, just sometimes, I even forget that she has cancer. Those are the types of moments you want to shoot for.

17

Avoid Transferring Your Fear to Your Dog

Jane Luba

While dogs live in the moment, they still can sense when their owners are sad or afraid. In many ways, your dog is a reflection of you. If you are afraid, your dog feels afraid.

This next tip comes from Jane Luba of Centreville, Virginia, owner of Oscar, the "happiest dog in the world," according to Jane. At ten years old, Oscar was diagnosed with mast cell cancer and lived another three exuberant years. She credits the removal of fear from her dog's environment as equally important to the medical treatment Oscar received.

As thinking beings, humans are both blessed and cursed. We can reason and problem solve, resulting in the incredible technological advances we see in the world today. But, on the other hand, we worry and fret about things that may or may not happen, causing incredible amounts of unnecessary stress. Dogs, on the other hand, only really react to the present moment, whether avoiding imminent danger or relishing in the bliss of their owner's attention.

So when you combine the worrisome tendencies of humans with a cancer diagnosis of their beloved best friend, there is an obvious conflict. In other words, the fear of losing your dog to cancer can do more harm than good.

Unlike humans, dogs don't fear cancer. Many times, they don't even know that they are sick. This is the quality that many humans admire the most about dogs—the ability to truly live in the moment—and why I believe dogs are man's best friend. In many ways, dogs are like innocent children subscribing to an "ignorance is bliss" approach to life.

Remember that while dogs do live in the moment, they still can sense when their owners are sad or afraid. In many ways, your dog is a reflection of you. If you are afraid, your dog feels afraid. And if your dog is feeling afraid, this means that he is stressed, which lessens his chances of winning the cancer battle.

To that end, don't transfer your fear to your dog. Don't cry in front of them, and don't let them smell your fear. Easier said than done; I know this first hand. But it can be done. It starts by truly believing your dog will get better—this kind of attitude naturally starts to permeate your daily attitude and will be transferred to your dog. Of course, you also have to do something to help your dog heal physically. In most cases, believing alone won't get your dog to be cancer-free, but they do go hand in hand.

Just like in humans, stress causes a fight, flight, or freeze response in dogs, which releases the hormone cortisone into their bodies. This is a useful hormone for a true emergency, like being attacked by another dog, but chronic stress means a continual high level of cortisone, which does not bode well for an already compromised immune system, as in the case of a dog with cancer. So not transferring your fear to your dog is not just an airy-fairy concept. It has a real physical response in your animal.

In my case, Oscar, a happy-go-lucky Cockapoo, was diagnosed with a mast cell tumor on his back left foot. We had the tumor surgically removed and did radiation and chemotherapy. We gave him all the scientific tools he needed, but we also added something equally important: no stress. So I did my best to manage my fear and I believe it truly helped. Oscar would happily go to his regular oncology appointments without a worry in the world and, as a result, lived three more extremely happy years to the age of thirteen.

Use a Holistic Approach

Natalie Stemp

People often confuse "holistic" with "alternative," misjudging it as a polarized approach to Western medicine. A holistic approach is just the opposite. It is a complete system, bringing together the best of traditional and alternative approaches.

"Your dog has cancer" was not what Natalie and Stan Stemp hoped to hear on their wedding anniversary. Simon, their seven-year-old, movie-star-cute Black Lab mix had been off his game for a few weeks. On June 10, 2008, he was diagnosed with stage four lymphoma, which had compromised his liver and spleen. The veterinary oncologist explained the success rate of chemotherapy against lymphoma, but gave Simon six to nine months to live even with chemo and six weeks without it. They opted for a holistic approach, which they believe doubled Simon's life expectancy.

Simon was diagnosed with lymphoma, a systemic cancer that spreads fairly quickly via the lymphatic system. Because it affects the entire body, you cannot simply remove a tumor. You need a systemic approach.

People often confuse "holistic" with "alternative," misjudging it as a polarized approach to Western medicine. A holistic approach is just the opposite. It is a complete system, bringing together the best of traditional and alternative approaches. It is not Western or Eastern, but both. You need both to outwit the cancer.

My husband and I decided to attack Simon's cancer in every way possible with a comprehensive plan that fused Eastern and Western approaches. Our goal was to give Simon the best chance at overcoming cancer and resuming a happy, healthy life. To accomplish this, we needed to take advantage of all the tools at our disposal, and we needed to think outside of the box. We used traditional medicine and alternative therapies, including supplements, exercise, massage, and a nontoxic environment to fight his cancer.

We decided to use chemotherapy, because it has a solid success rate (with a life expectancy of a year for over 80 percent of the cases, depending on the stage) against lymphoma. Simon's protocol had two major side effects—weight loss due to the killing of large quantities of cancer cells (a good thing), and weight loss due to stomach upset (a bad thing). In essence, chemo is a poison that not only kills cancer cells, but also compromises healthy cells. As such, you need to find a way to make the host environment unsuitable for cancer cells while giving good cells the support they need to fight the cancer cells and tolerate chemo. How do you pull this off? Feed the body substances that the good cells need for battle, and remove substances that feed or potentially activate the cancer cells. This is where the Eastern part of the plan takes the stage supporting the Western part.

Through the Eastern approach, you examine diet to ensure the body gets the nutrients it needs through nutrition and supplements to remain strong and fight cancer. Simon's diet gave him the right kinds and pro-portions of protein, omega fatty acids, fiber, antioxidants, minerals, fat, and vitamins. This was key because Simon's liver and spleen were compromised, so we had to be cautious about his consumption of the fat, vitamins, and minerals that those organs ordinarily metabolize when healthy. There was no corn, wheat, or sugar in his diet, because cancer cells thrive on sugars and carbohydrates. To be sure to keep pesticides and additives out of his food and to keep full-strength nutrients in his food, we used only fresh, organic ingredients: yams, carrots, lentils, wild-caught salmon, spinach, and brown rice.

Simon is now in remission. We believe the powerful herbs and supple-ments he received were essential to his victory (to date) over cancer. To make sure no substances interfered with each other or his chemo, we carefully administered his regimen of ten or so antioxidants, enzymes, and other detoxifiers on a strict schedule. Most of these sup-plements supported the immune system, heart, thyroid, bones, liver, and normal cell division and production, all of which are weakened by cancer and chemo. I believe our comprehensive plan has nearly doubled Simon's life expectancy and has helped him return to his happy, silly self.

Remove Stress from Your Dog's Life

Aimee Quemuel

Reducing the stress your dog experiences helps focus his or her energy on fighting the cancer, not the stress.

Keeping your dog relaxed and stress free is another important tool in the fight against cancer. Reducing the stress your dog experiences helps focus his or her energy on fighting the cancer, not the stress.

As the keeper of your dog, you likely know exactly what stresses them out. For Cody, it was three things: my other dog CJ, being separated from me, and going to the veterinarian.

CJ, my other Golden Retriever, did not come into our lives until Cody was almost nine years old. By this time, Cody was a mature Golden Retriever that was used to my focused attention. For the first seven months, Cody would not even look at CJ. And when Cody was diagnosed with cancer, CJ was still a very hyper two-year-old puppy. CJ did not know that Cody was sick. He simply wanted to play. But I knew that CJ's constant pestering was not supporting Cody's fight against dog cancer. So I made sure that Cody had plenty of alone time. My boyfriend at the time would take CJ, and I would take Cody. This way, both dogs got the attention they needed, and Cody got the undistracted alone time he needed to heal.

Cody was one of the most well behaved dogs I have ever seen. But he did have one major fault—insane separation anxiety. He had to be by my side and when he was not, he would bark incessantly. I was lucky in that I worked from home so I was able to have him with me at most times. When he was first diagnosed, I canceled all plans and all vacations. I had friends come visit me at home instead of going out. And for Thanksgiving, despite being the only family member in San Francisco, most of my family members travelled to me so that Cody and I would not be alone. Because I was told his condition was so dire, I refused to leave his side. But after the five months, Cody's condition improved, and I had to find a way to bring some normalcy back into my life. So I slowly started to leave—at first for twenty minutes, then for an hour, and then for a few hours. Whether gone twenty minutes or a few hours, I always placed his favorite toys around him. I also left soothing music on and gave him dehydrated chicken treats to distract him as I slipped away.

The last stress, and probably a pretty common one among all dogs, was visiting the veterinarian office. Cody would literally start shaking the moment he realized where we were. And with his cancer condition, we were seemingly going to the veterinarian on a weekly basis. His panic attacks surely were not good for his health. As such, I started asking the veterinarian to come to me; not a house call, but to the back of my car to draw blood or to do a routine exam. At first, my veterinarian looked at me like I was crazy. But I insisted. I told her that it is too stressful for Cody and because he felt safe in the car, I would prefer if she came to the car to perform any tests or exams. She did it, and Cody was able to get the necessary tests without the stress.

Stimulate the Lymphatic System

Aimee Quemuel and Jill Spencer

The lymphatic system is so important to your dog's health that if movement stopped entirely, your dog would die in a matter of hours.

The lymphatic system is comprised of a network of vessels and hundreds of nodes that run through your dog's entire body, the tonsils, thymus, and the spleen and works in conjunction with the circulatory system and the immune system. As detailed on the Web site Lymphomation.org, http://www.lymphomation.org/lymphatic.htm, the lymphatic system performs these important functions:

- It aids the immune system by destroying pathogens and filtering waste.

- It removes excess fluid, waste, debris, dead blood cells, pathogens, cancer cells, and toxins from the cells and the tissue spaces between them.

- It works with the circulatory system to deliver nutrients, oxygen, and hormones from the blood to the cells.

- It delivers important protein molecules that are created by cells in the tissues that are too large to be carried by the circulatory system.

The lymphatic system is so important to your dog's health that if the movement stopped entirely, your dog would die in a matter of hours. However, unlike the circulatory system that is moved by the heart, the lymphatic system does not have its own pump. Movement is dependent upon muscle expansion and contraction. In other words, it only moves as much as your dog does.

So if the lymphatic system moves toxins out of the body such as cancer cells, and if you have control over how quickly the system moves, then it comes to reason that moving the lymphatic system as quickly as possible is another key tool to fighting dog cancer and is the essence of this next rule: move your dog's lymphatic system.

The most common way to move the lymphatic system is through exercise. This was the choice for Jill Spencer, owner of RCi (pronounced R-C), and author of Rule 30, Boost Their Immunity with Antioxidants. RCi survived her cancer for thirty-four months, having no tumor removal, chemo, or radiation treatments.

One of RCi's favorite things to do was to run and play tug-of-war with a flattened football with the Spencers' two Rat Terriers, Reeci and Riki. In addition to her play sessions, RCi went for two-mile walks four to six days a week. Depending on your dog's condition, exercising your pet could be a simple walk around the yard, jogging the neighborhood, playing ball or Frisbee, taking him for a swim, or working with him on training exercises; teaching your pet new skills is very motivating and stimulating for them.

The bottom line is that exercise on a consistent basis is definitely a benefit to your pet's health regardless of cancer. It keeps your pet active, healthier, and happier. In addition, exercising with your pet is a special bond-developing moment and time where you are establishing your pack leadership with them.

According to Jill, "All you have to do is look into their eyes when you mention it is time to go for a walk or go play ball and you see the sparkle in their eyes and happy body language, which are positive indicators how special this time for them is with you. So keep exercise as an everyday ritual not only for their health, but also as a relationship builder."

But what if exercise is not an option? What if your dog's ability to exercise is prohibited by his current condition? Maybe he just had surgery or maybe he is just too weak at the moment. Fortunately, there are other ways besides exercise to move the lymphatic system.

Acupuncture, massage, and just plain old brushing all move the lymphatic system. However, keep in mind that some experts warn that acupuncture might stimulate and reawaken cancer in dogs in remission. Whichever method you decide on, the point is, the more you move your dog's body, whether through exercise or touch, the more your dog's lymphatic system moves —and removing poisons and toxins from your dog's body is definitely a requirement in supporting wellness and fighting cancer.

Remove Toxins from Your Dog's Body

Rosemary Levesque

It is critical to remove the toxins from your dog's body (and your own) to help win the fight against cancer.

After nearly a lifetime of battling diabetes, Rosemary's twelve-and-a-half-year-old Yellow Lab, Ginger, was diagnosed with hemangiosarcoma, an incurable blood cancer that typically metastasizes to the lungs, heart, liver, and spleen. Using a combination of surgery, detoxification, supplements, and energy healing, Ginger lived sixteen additional healthy months with her family in Portland, Oregon—more than fourteen months beyond her expected survival date.

Studies have shown that many chronic conditions such as cancer or neurological challenges can result from an overload of heavy metals, pesticides, flame retardants, and other toxins in our environment. These toxins burden our systems. That is why I believe it is critical to remove the toxins from your dog's body (and your own) to help win the fight against cancer. When the obstacles to health are taken away, the body can then experience the benefits of proper functioning and good health.

I first discovered liquid zeolite, Natural Cellular Defense, in May 2006. It is safe and the most effective way to remove toxins. I knew that we needed to be active in our health, and I could think of other people who would want liquid zeolite too. With a firm belief that an ounce of prevention is worth a pound of cure, I decided to start with the "minimum" dose for my family members, including Ginger, to help them remove the unavoidable toxins that we are exposed to on a daily basis.

Insulin-dependent since the age of seven, Ginger was already on a healthy raw diet to help regulate her blood sugar. After about a week of using liquid zeolite, Ginger passed a purple, slimy stool that I thought was a sign of detox. What I saw might have actually been evidence of growths being expelled from the body. She had an unexplained cough that disappeared too. Ginger seemed to have a little more energy during that time, but we didn't know what was really happening. Admittedly, we were inconsistent at giving her regular doses of liquid zeolite after the first month.

On September 20, 2006, Ginger collapsed. Her blood sugar was high and dangerous for her. Ginger couldn't stand and we brought her to our local emergency hospital where she was diagnosed with a ruptured spleen caused by hemangiosarcoma.

Despite the grim outlook from the doctors—sixteen to sixty days with surgery, immediate death without—we opted for emergency surgery to remove her spleen and stop the massive bleeding. I felt in my heart that we had the ultimate weapon and that Ginger would make it. By this time I had learned that many people and animals in a health crisis such as Ginger's had overcome the cancer beast. We could too. We had hope in a bottle.

Looking back, I realize that the preventative detoxification dose I was giving her was also helping her in her fight. During her four days in ICU, Ginger received ten drops of zeolite every fifteen minutes around the clock. At home we continued with a high therapeutic dose of one hundred drops per day. We were in a race for her life. Not only was she able to survive surgery at her old age and health condition, we saw her thrive.

Remarkably, in the following weeks, Ginger's dependence on insulin lessened. It seemed that her diabetes was reversing. Indeed, even the scar tissue from her injection site was gone. There were no signs of cancer, no signs of arthritis, and she had energy like a puppy.

Ginger passed from old age just shy of her fourteenth birthday. Cancer-free without chemo, I firmly believe that high doses of liquid zeolite gave us more quality time with my Ginger—sixteen more happy and healthy months. Her lesson for us is clear: don't wait for cancer to strike you and your family, as we never know what diseases we can prevent by making good decisions about our health now.

22 Keep Detailed Notes

Laurie Kaplan

The simple notations in your log could help you get a repeat episode under control quickly.

Laurie Kaplan, author of Help Your Dog Fight Cancer, *recommends that you keep a log of your dog's journey. Laurie's dog Bullet was diagnosed with lymphoma and lived for four-plus years past diagnosis.*

Keeping track of your treatments and notable events is critical in your fight. The simple notations in your log could help you get a repeat episode under control quickly. Veterinarians you consult may ask for information such as when you started giving your dog a particular medication or supplement, at what doses, and how he responded. If your log contains the answers, it will help the doctor make the most effective recommendations without delay.

Try to update your notes as soon as possible to ensure their accuracy. The longer you wait, the more likely you will forget an important aspect of your treatment plan.

Some suggested items to include in your log are:

- Medications and supplements given
- Any change in diet
- Any changes in eating, urination, and defecation habits or mood
- Names and dates of treatments
- Side effects and reactions
- All attempts to counteract side effects

- What worked and what didn't

- How long it took for the remedy to resolve the problem

- Who recommended the remedy

- Secondary illnesses

Keeping a log or journal of events during your dog's cancer journey will also be therapeutic for you! Keeping Bullet's log up to date gave me a sense of confidence. I was aware of and had a record of the history of events, every side effect and remedy, medication, and supplement and its effect. If a health issue reoccurred I would know quickly how to resolve it. I could look at my log and say, "I have been here before, and I know how to address this issue." Thanks to the log, I was able to improve and fine-tune Bullet's diet and supplement regimen very easily and request changes in the chemo protocol.

Imagine if your experiences could help other dogs with cancer! By sharing your detailed notes, you may very well help others fighting for their dogs' lives. In fact, I would have been hard pressed to provide or remember much of the information in my book without the log that I kept for Bullet.

Before I wrote the book outlining Bullet's cancer journey, I was recruited by Bullet's veterinarian to help his other clients who had dogs with cancer. I consulted one family at a time, reviewing their dog's treatment protocol and home care regimen. I referred constantly to my copious notes. With half of all dogs likely to get cancer, I knew I had to find a better way to get Bullet's story out there, and this was my motivation for writing the book.

Aimee Quemuel, the author of this book, offers a wonderful tool for keeping such a log. Fight Dog Cancer http://www.fightdogcancer.com, is a free online service where you can tell your dog's story and create a log of your dog's cancer journey all in one place and accessible to anyone online. In addition to using Fight Dog Cancer's online logbook for the benefit of your dog, you can also help others benefit from your experiences to help their own dogs. Your veterinarian can access the information easily too, just let the doctor know that your log is at that web site.

23 Just Get Them to Eat

Kristine Tanzillo

Having something new to look forward to really kept Sheldon going.

At fourteen and three-quarters years old, Sheldon was diagnosed with stomach cancer and given six weeks to live. Quickly disintegrating and down to a svelte fifteen pounds (from thirty pounds), Kristine thought it was time to say goodbye. But a fallen scoop of ice cream on the floor became the catalyst that bought Sheldon sixteen more months.

Months leading up to the cancer diagnosis, Sheldon had been vomiting, which quickly became a daily occurrence. The veterinarian put him on a series of medications to help with the nausea, but they ironically seemed to make things worse. After Sheldon's diagnosis, we took him home and stopped all of his anti-nausea medicine—he was just throwing them up anyway. He refused to eat and was nearly half of his original weight. We thought it was the end and were just waiting for his time to come.

But one night, something miraculous happened. We dropped ice cream on the floor, and, to our surprise, Sheldon ate it. And so it began—a sixteen-month journey with food. After the ice-cream incident, we started offering him soft foods such as yogurt and scrambled eggs and, of course, ice cream. Ice cream became a nightly ritual between Sheldon and my husband. We then stepped it up to turkey, grilled cheese, and vegetables. We figured it didn't matter what he ate at this point as long he received some nourishment. When he stopped drinking water, we offered him sweet tea and Coke, which he became quite fond of.

Sometime near Christmas (about eight weeks after the diagnosis), he stopped throwing up as much and began to show signs of life. Because he was so frail he couldn't eat much at one time, he had to eat often. We offered him food when we ate breakfast, lunch, and dinner. His appetite slowly picked up and he started eating on a regular basis again. We started a routine of feeding him three times a day—basically every time we ate a meal. For breakfast we started giving him homemade waffles, pancakes, or eggs. For lunch he received turkey or a grilled cheese sandwich. And for dinner he ate what we ate, including vegetables. And at 8:00 p.m. every evening, he began circling the kitchen and standing in front of the refrigerator for his nightly bowl of vanilla ice cream.

Within three to four months of his cancer diagnosis, he appeared normal. He gained weight, was eating regularly and was socializing with the family again. We decided to continue the feeding routine. His cancer was still prevalent, but for unknown reasons it wasn't as debilitating as it had been. He stopped vomiting almost completely; when he did vomit, we offered him Sprite or some other mild carbonated drink to soothe his stomachache.

We continued this regime for a year and four months. We celebrated his sixteenth birthday with a large vanilla ice cream cake from Baskin Robbins. He received a piece of this cake every night for almost a week. About two weeks after his sixteenth birthday, Sheldon passed away in his sleep. He had a stroke, which left him impaired on one side.

We honestly don't know what took him from the brink of death to life for another year and four months. I later found out that protein and fats are thought to be cancer-fighting foods for dogs—both of which were included in Sheldon's daily diet. In addition, I think having something new to look forward to really kept Sheldon going. Whatever it was, we thank God for the extra time we had with him. And we are most thankful we didn't listen to those who told us to put him down when we received the diagnosis.

Know What Goes into Your Dog

Aimee Quemuel and Robin Barbosa

It doesn't take much research to find out just how detrimental some commercial dog foods are to our dogs...especially if they are fighting cancer.

As the saying goes, "You are what you eat." The same holds true for our dogs. Every component and process in your dog's body starts with what they eat. What you feed your dog is a critical component to his fight against cancer, as many owners of dogs fighting cancer can attest to. By knowing exactly what goes into your dog, you are able to better track what is working and what is not.

The day that I found out about Cody's cancer, I immediately put him on a cancer diet. I kept copious notes. I scoured the Internet and consulted with numerous veterinarians and fellow dog owners to come up with a diet that Cody not only loved, but that also helped drive his cancer into remission. While there are many recipes out there, they all seem to have a few things in common: high protein, low carbohydrates, and high fat.

Research shows that animals with cancer have an altered carbohydrate metabolism, so a diet that is low in carbohydrates and contains high-quality proteins and fish oil as the primary fat source, best meets the needs of the animal cancer patient. I also monitored what treats he was allowed to eat, which in Cody's case was only dehydrated chicken jerky. I had a hard time finding organic ones, so I made my own. Time-consuming for sure, but I knew at all times exactly what went into Cody, which made it easier to shift things if Cody's health was declining.

Robin Barbosa, whose Beagle, Disnay, survived six and a half years with mast cell cancer, attributes Disnay's survival to the raw vegetable diet she received, consisting of grated carrots, cauliflower, and broccoli stalks with chicken and flaxseed oil.

It doesn't take much research to find out just how detrimental some commercial dog foods are to our dogs...especially if they are fighting cancer.

In my opinion, a home-cooked meal using organic ingredients is the "Holy Grail." This ensures that you know exactly what is going into your beloved dog. Some experts recommend you feed them raw meat, others recommend it cooked. While I opted for raw, I think it is more important to use a good quality animal-based protein. Also keep in mind that if your pet is undergoing chemotherapy or radiation, cooked food is recommended.

The downside to home-cooked/prepared food is it is more expensive than cheap kibble and time-consuming. However, if you make the food in batches, that can save time. I have also heard of people doing co-ops, in which they bought their organic dog meat in bulk to save money. Sunday was my dog food day in which I would make a week's worth of Cody's food.

If you do have to feed some commercial dog food, make sure to read your dog food label! The first ingredient on the list should be some type of meat (and not a by-product or meal). There are more and more grain-free diets such as Stella and Chewy's, http://www.stellaandchewys.com/. And if you must feed commercial kibble, supplement it with an animal protein source such as eggs, sardines, hamburger, or chicken.

25 Feed Enzyme-Rich Food

Aimee Quemuel

If you want to do everything you can to help your dog fight cancer, then feeding an enzyme-rich diet and enzyme supplements is highly recommended.

Digestive enzymes help break down food so that nutrients can be absorbed by your dog's body. They are found in natural, uncooked foods (like raw meat and finely grated vegetables) and are destroyed at temperatures above 118 degrees Fahrenheit. They are a critical part of your dog's digestive system and, in general, are important for any dog's health and longevity, especially older dogs. For your dog fighting cancer, they are vital.

A healthy digestive system improves your dog's ability to fight off cancer and prevents the "wasting away" effect often associated with cancer. Most cancer dogs die from secondary organ failure, not the cancer itself, so anything you do to keep vital organs strong will only bode well for your fight. If you want to do everything you can to help your dog fight cancer, then feeding an enzyme-rich diet and enzyme supplements is highly recommended.

As your dog eats, the pancreas secretes enzymes to help with the digestion process. The pancreas is so vital that insufficient secretion of digestive enzymes by the pancreas leads to starvation, even if your dog is consuming adequate quantities of high quality food. Feeding enzyme-rich, uncooked foods aids the digestive system so your dog's pancreas and digestive system in general don't have to work as hard to break down food. In addition, enzyme-rich foods help break down food faster, which means they are not only absorbed faster, but also there is less wear and tear on your dog's body. On the flip side, eating processed or cooked foods means the body has to do all the work, causing undue stress. Plus, nutrition is absorbed at a much slower and lower rate.

Even if your dog eats enzyme-rich natural foods, adding supplemental digestive enzymes doesn't hurt. It can only help as the energy used to digest food could be diverted to help fight off the cancer instead.

Adding digestive enzymes to your dog's diet is quite easy. As mentioned, using enzyme-rich foods such as raw meat and finely grated vegetables is the ideal; however, if you must feed processed or cooked food, you can easily add a digestive enzyme supplement.

To aid digestion even more, I would "pre-digest" Cody's food by adding supplemental enzymes to his food prior to serving so that the enzymes started working on the food before it entered his body. If you are using dry food, you will need to add a little warm water to activate the enzymes. But remember the warm water you add or the food can't be above 118 degrees or you kill the enzymes.

When I first started on the dog cancer journey with Cody, I used Prozyme, an enzyme blend made especially for dogs. Later, since I also took digestive enzymes for my own health, I gave Cody the same human blend I used. There are plenty of choices available, but keep in mind that digestive enzymes are specialized in that they will only work on specific food types so you will want to make sure whatever brand you use has the following:

- Amylase, which breaks down carbohydrates

- Cellulase, which breaks down vegetables and fibers

- Lipase, which breaks down fats

- Protease, which breaks down proteins

The final point to consider is that many dogs fighting cancer are likely taking an arsenal of additional supplements. The supplements, in theory, are meant to attack the cancer in one form or another; however, it is also makes the body, particularly the liver, work harder.

While digestive enzymes don't help metabolize supplements themselves, they provide your dog's body a valuable break so that energy can be focused elsewhere, such as metabolizing of supplements aimed squarely at fighting the cancer.

26 Stay Away from Grains

Aimee Quemuel

The most important rule for feeding a dog with cancer is to stay away from grains such as corn, wheat, and rice. Most commercial dog food companies and even dog biscuit manufacturers use grains as the main ingredient because it is cheap so they can make a bigger profit. So even if the food meets the minimum protein requirements, if the food contains high-levels of grains, then it is bad for your dog—especially those fighting cancer.

Here's why: Cancer utilizes carbohydrates for fuel. And grains are carbohydrates. Plus dogs did not evolve as grain eaters—they are primarily meat eaters. They simply do not produce the enzymes necessary to digest grains. So the fewer carbohydrates in the form of grains you feed your dog, the less fuel the cancer has to spread in your dog's body.

Historically speaking, a wild dog's diet contains almost no grains. And they never eat cooked grain. They may eat some grains via the intestinal tracts of their prey, but it is partially digested.

In contrast, today's modern dog eats mostly grains. Many veterinarians blame grain-based diets for diabetes, digestive problems, and cancer. Cody, unfortunately, ate dry kibble his entire life, so he was not only subjected to an "unnatural" diet, but also possibly exposed to two very dangerous carcinogens: aflatoxin and acrylamide.

Aflatoxin is a mold that grows on corn, rice, and other grains. According to Wikipedia, "Aflatoxins are toxic and among the most carcinogenic substances known." For a dog already suffering with cancer, such a toxin could be deadly.

Another carcinogen found in grain-based foods is acrylamide. Acrylamide is a natural by-product that forms when certain carbohydrate-rich foods are fried, baked, or roasted at high temperatures above 120 degrees Celcius. Acrylamide cannot be created by boiling foods, and raw foods contain very little detectable amounts. Baking, microwaving, frying, or deep-frying will produce acrylamide, and overcooking foods may produce large amounts of acrylamide. French fries and potato chips contain the highest concentrations, but acrylamide occurs in breads and breakfast cereals as well.

Research shows that acrylamide causes cancer in rats when administered orally in high-dose experiments and increased tumors in the nervous system, oral cavity peritoneum, thyroid gland, mammary gland, uterus, and clitoris. The U.S. Environmental Protection Agency (EPA) has set the "safe level" for human consumption at almost zero, with the maximum safe level in drinking water set at 0.5 parts per billion.[iii]

Considering how common these carcinogens are and given the fact that cancer cells thrive on carbohydrates, it is prudent for dogs fighting cancer to avoid grains altogether.

There have not been tests done on pet foods, but any processed foods that contain carbohydrates—especially those extruded at high temperatures, like grain-based kibble, or canned under high heat and pressure—pose a risk.

All Proteins Are Not Created Equal

Aimee Quemuel

In the case of a dog fighting cancer, quality and quantity are equally important.

I have always been an avid label reader. I always made sure that the dog food I bought for my dogs met the minimum requirements as set forth by the Association of American Feed Control Officials (AAFCO). I had assumed that this stamp of approval meant that it was safe for my dog and, just like the label said, would enable my family member to live a long, healthy life. But it wasn't until Cody was diagnosed with cancer that I discovered the truth of the matter: all ingredients, including the protein count, are not created equal.

A dog with cancer is building a lot of new tissue. New tissue requires protein. If the right amount of quality protein is not present in your dog's diet, then the body will rob it from organs or muscles. This is what causes the "wasting away" effect, which, if left unchecked, can cause secondary complications and sometimes death.

But not all proteins are created equally. In the case of a dog fighting cancer, quality and quantity are equally important.

Remember the 2007 pet food recall? That was caused by melamine, which was used to artificially increase the protein content of the food. Melamine—which is a commercial by-product—is used to make plastics and cleaning products, and is **not** approved for use as an ingredient in human or animal food. While the dog food containing the melamine had the proper quantity of protein according to tests, the quality was obviously not up to par, and it is thought that nearly two thousand cats and more than two thousand two hundred dogs died as a result. Obviously, this is an extreme example, but the point is clear: you have to make sure the quality of the protein is up to snuff.

Beyond quality protein, using animal protein over plant-based protein is also important. Dogs are meat eaters. They have always eaten meat. Dogs thrive on meat-based diets. High-quality **animal** protein such as chicken or beef, preferably organic, is highly recommended for your dog fighting cancer.

Using organic reduces the amount of pesticides and toxins that your already ailing dog needs to deal with. Animals raised organically are not fed antibiotics and not given bovine human growth hormone (rBGH) or other artificial drugs. They are also not allowed to eat genetically modified foods.

In addition, certified organic meats means synthetic pesticides and fertilizers are not used on the food or land the animals are raised on. Residues of persistent chemicals such as DDT, PCBs, dioxin, and many pesticides concentrate in animal fat. Eating organic meat reduces your exposure to these chemicals.

Lastly, the words "free range," and "ranch raised" are clues that the animals were raised in a more humane way. Their diets tend to be more well rounded, and the animals are not confined and spend time outdoors in the fresh air, which means the animals are likely more healthy than their caged counterparts.

While for most dogs, protein should make up the majority of their diets, it is important to note that this is not always the case. You should always customize diet based on your dog's specific needs. For example, protein is hard on the kidneys, so if your dog has kidney issues, you will need to tailor your diet to his or her needs and feed as little protein as possible.

28 Omega-6 Bad, Omega-3 Good

Aimee Quemuel

Dry kibble is loaded with Omega-6, which, in excess, has been linked to a plethora of diseases, including cancer.

Despite a long history in the field of marketing, I fell prey to the pet food industry's promises of health and vitality and unknowingly fed my beloved Cody one of the worst possible foods: dry kibble. Commercial dog food, especially dry kibble, is loaded with Omega-6, which, in excess, has been linked to a plethora of diseases, including cancer. I personally believe that Cody's poor diet was a key contributing factor to his development of cancer. But, by the same token, if your dog is still with you, you still have a chance. Act now. Evaluate the causes later. Time is most definitely of the essence.

Omega-3 and Omega-6 are considered essential fatty acids (EFAs). They are essential to human health, but are not produced by the body. For this reason, they must be obtained from food. Just like humans, dogs need to have a certain ratio of Omega-3 to Omega-6 fatty acids in their diet.

The exact ideal ratio for dogs has yet to be determined, but most veterinarians believe the ratio is somewhere between 5:1 and 10:1 (Omega-6: Omega-3). We do know, however, that most dogs have an Omega-6/Omega-3 imbalance. Here is why:

Just like the typical human diet, most commercial dog foods are rich in Omega-6, but lack Omega-3, which is why most dogs have a heavily imbalanced ratio of Omega-6 fatty acids to Omega-3 fatty acids. Omega-6 can be found in virtually all processed foods including commercial dog foods, vegetable cooking oils, soybean oil, sunflower oil, canola oil, and corn oil (but not olive oil). Despite all the promises of longevity and concern for the health of your dog, the bottom line is that the dog food industry is a multi-billion dollar industry mostly concerned with their profit margins. And guess what? You guessed it—the cheapest ingredients are the ones packed with Omega-6 fatty acids.

When there is an excess of Omega-6 in the body, bad things start to happen. Omega-6 increases inflammation, and since inflammation has long been associated with cancer, it makes sense that the more inflammation, the harder it will be for your dog to recover from cancer. On the flip side, Omega-3 reduces inflammation. So it makes sense that increasing Omega-3 will help your dog's battle against cancer.

When Cody was first diagnosed, one of the first things I did was start him on megadoses of fish oil to get his fatty acids in balance. I gave him 1000 mg per 20 lbs of body weight per day, which, at seventy-five pounds, meant he got four 1000 mg capsules per day. Since it is nearly impossible to give your dog too much Omega-3 fatty acids, I also fed him Omega-3 rich foods such as sardines, menhaden, mackerel, and salmon. Omega-3 is also abundant in walnuts, flaxseed, and green leafy vegetables, but I had a harder time feeding those foods to Cody, so I stuck to the "stinky fishes" that had the additional benefit of enticing him to eat, since my boy was a pretty picky eater. Some veterinarians recommend even higher doses—up to 18 grams per 60 lbs, which is about 15-20 human dosage capsules.

One word of caution, though, is that some research points to Omega-3 as a blood thinner, which should be taken into consideration if your dog is going to have surgery.

29 Give and Use Purified Water

Aimee Quemuel

Of the 141 unregulated contaminants detected in water supplies between 1998 and 2003, fifty-two are linked to cancer.

I always drank filtered water, but for some reason it never dawned on me that I should do the same for my dogs. I guess I just figured that the higher powers (the people that regulate such things as water), would warn us if tap water really posed a danger to our animals and us. But boy was I wrong.

According to the Environmental Protection Agency (EPA), "Your water supplier must notify you by newspaper, mail, radio, TV, or hand-delivery if your water doesn't meet EPA or state standards or if there is a waterborne disease emergency."[iv] I think the key term here is "disease emergency." So, essentially, if it is not going to make you sick immediately, they don't have to tell you what is really in the water.

A December 2005 analysis of more than 22 million tap water quality tests, most of which were required under the federal Safe Drinking Water Act, found that water suppliers across the U.S. detected 260 contaminants in public tap water.[v] Of the 141 unregulated contaminants detected in water supplies between 1998 and 2003, 52 are linked to cancer, 41 to reproductive toxicity, 36 to developmental toxicity, and 16 to immune system damage. Water contaminated with 83 agricultural pollutants, including pesticides and fertilizer ingredients, flows through the taps of over 200 million Americans in 41 states.

The problem is not your water company's failure to warn you of the dangers of tap water, it is the EPA's failure to establish enforceable health standards for tap water contaminants. Of the 260 contaminants detected in tap water from 42 states, the EPA has set enforceable health limits (called Maximum Contaminant Levels, or MCLs) for only 114, and, for five others, the Agency has set non-enforceable goals called secondary standards. The other 141 remaining chemicals (as of the 2005 analysis) continued to contaminate water served to 195,257,000 people in 22,614 communities in 42 states.

The bottom line is that I was not going to wait for the EPA to start regulating the safety of our water. My boy was sick, and I was going to change one of the key elements that sustained him on a daily basis: his water.

I started him on the filtered and bottled water immediately. I selected one that also had electrolytes and minerals as well to make sure Cody was truly getting the hydration he needed. I also installed a water filtration system in my shower where Cody was given a bath. Just like humans, a dog's largest organ is the skin and I wanted to make sure when I bathed Cody that nasty tap water was not getting into his system.

As a side note, I have become more educated about the dangers of plastic bottles and now only drink filtered water that comes in glass bottles from Mountain Valley Spring, http://www.mountainvalleyspring.com/, as does my 5-year-old Golden, CJ, who is still with me.

Boost Immunity with Antioxidants

Jill Spencer

We have always been convinced in the use of antioxidants and supplements for health benefits, (antioxidants neutralize free radicals), so we decided to try a regimen of supplements that are high in antioxidants on RCi for her cancer.

At just six years old, Jill and Mike Spencer's Doberman Pinscher, RCi (pronounced R-C), was diagnosed with cancer of the connective tissue. Jill decided to use a completely all-natural approach, which included a supplemental mix high in antioxidants such as spirulina, chlorella, millet, flax seed and L-glutamine. The results were beyond all expectations—RCi survived thirty-four quality months!

On January 2003, our beloved six-year-old, female Doberman, RCi, was diagnosed with fibrosarcoma (cancer of connective tissue). This was confirmed via a biopsy report from a university pathology lab. Before the biopsy, RCi's tumor was the size of a marble. During the biopsy procedure a core sample of the tumor was taken, which aggravated the tumor, and, within days, the marble-sized tumor grew to a fist size (approximately 8–9 cm) protruding from her upper left ribcage.

A veterinary oncologist gave RCi two to three months to live with no treatment, or an 80 percent chance to live a "possible" year after radical treatment that included surgery to remove the tumor and four ribs and radiation treatment every week for ten weeks at a university 125 miles away. We decided tumor removal and radiation treatments were NOT an option, simply because it was too radical. Cracking a rib is painful, so can you imagine the pain associated with removing four of them and having reconstructive surgery of the ribcage? RCi would have had to endure a great deal of physical and emotional trauma, and her quality of life would have been significantly compromised. The worst part was our inability to explain to RCi why we would be putting her through a distressing ordeal like this.

We have always been convinced in the use of antioxidants and supplements for health benefits, (antioxidants neutralize free radicals), so we decided to try a regimen of supplements that are high in antioxidants on RCi for her cancer. Originally, we had consulted with supplement experts, Patti and Ed Bishop, General Nutrition Center (GNC) franchise owners, because of our mother/mother-in-law's diagnosis of stage three/four ovarian cancer in September 2002. Patti is a survivor of bladder cancer, and she told us what she did to boost her immune system to help fight her cancer after tumor removal and before monthly treatments.

We also researched via the Internet, read various independent studies, and talked with herbal experts to create this antioxidant-supplemental mix that included spirulina, chlorella, millet, flax seed and L-Glutamine—all aimed at helping boost RCi's immune system to fight against the cancer. In addition, we changed RCi's diet and made sure she was exercised on a regular basis.

In the thirty-four months from RCi's cancer diagnosis of January 2003, our decision to go with a high antioxidant-supplemental route was truly an amazing journey. Her tumor, which was a fist-sized mass protruding from her ribcage, was suddenly reduced in size, but best of all, RCi's health was as robust as ever. RCi's favorite thing to do was to puncture footballs, run around with them, and play tug-of-war with our two Rat Terriers, Reeci and Riki, which she did until the day she left us. In addition, she went for two-mile walks, four to six days a week.

We had over 1,020 days with RCi surviving her cancer, having no tumor removal, and no chemo or radiation treatments. Each day, I would look into her eyes and see life dancing in them and this is what brought joy to my heart. She simply amazed us and everyone she came in contact with, so we decided to offer the same antioxidant-supplemental mixture to other dog owners at A'Dobe Angel, http://www.adobeangel.com. We named it APA Immune Booster because of its properties of algae, plant enzymes, and amino acid. RCi got thirty-four months of quality life, and we credit it all to using supplements high in antioxidants. RCi's paw print is forever in our hearts.

Supplements Are Powerful Medicines

Taimi Dunn Gorman

While I personally used medicinal mushrooms to fight Liwu's cancer, there are lots of supplements touted to fight dog cancer.

In December of 2007, at eleven years old, Taimi Dunn Gorman's Chow, Liwu (pronounced lee-woo), was diagnosed with liver cancer. His tumors were so large that they pressed his organs to one side. The doctor said there was nothing they could do. Despite some traditional cancer medications (no chemo) along with his Rimadyl for arthritis pain, he began to deteriorate. Desperate, Taimi got on the Internet and stumbled upon a mushroom-based supplement that she credits for giving her eighteen more months with her beloved dog Liwu.

When Liwu was eleven years old in December 2007, I took him for his annual exam. As the veterinarian felt around, he discovered the tumors. His tumors were so large that they pressed his internal organs to one side. Since the liver is a vital organ, surgery was not an option. The veterinarian gave him a few weeks or perhaps a month or two, if we were lucky. We took him home and waited for the inevitable. Two months later, around February 2008, Liwu started to deteriorate. He lost his energy. He got scabs on his stomach that wouldn't heal. He lost his spark. I thought it was the end.

Desperate, I got on the Internet and stumbled upon a mushroom-based supplement made by a company called Aloha Medicinals. Knowing that medicinal mushrooms have long been used to heal immune-based diseases, I decided to give it a shot.

Although it was expensive, I continued to give Liwu his pills daily. After all, Liwu was my gift—my loyal dog that had been a part of my life for over a decade. There was no cost too high to give my beloved friend a dignified and quality end of life.

To my surprise, and within days, he began to perk up. He got his energy back. The wounds on his stomach healed. He started to act like his old self. Nothing else had changed—just the addition of the mushroom supplement.

True to his nature, Liwu hung in there, living a good life for a total of eighteen months post his diagnosis. Until the day he died at home with my husband by his side, he was still able to walk up and down the stairs to the dog door and do his rounds in the backyard. I completely credit his extra year of *quality* life to the mushroom-based supplement.

Interestingly, he waited to die until I was in Hawaii on vacation. They say animals do that to spare their masters from the pain of their departure. Even until the very end, Liwu was protecting me.

When he passed away, I donated the extra medicine to my veterinarian, who now recommends it to others with incurable cancer.

While I personally used medicinal mushrooms to fight Liwu's cancer, there are lots of supplements touted to fight dog cancer. You have to do the research to find one that makes sense for you and your dog. And you need to make sure that the supplements you include as part of your treatment plan won't have an adverse effect. Just don't discount supplements as powerful medicine to help your dog fight cancer. They worked for Liwu. They gave me another year to give him extra attention and another year to say goodbye.

32 Give Fresh Air

Aimee Quemuel

Many of our dogs are spending the majority of their lives indoors breathing in the same dirty indoor air that we are.

I was fortunate enough to live close to the beach and was able to take Cody on daily walks to the beach for some fresh air therapy. In addition, I made sure he spent as much time as possible outdoors and, weather permitting, would work on my laptop outdoors with Cody by my side. However, I, like many others, had to put my desk time in, which required being indoors. Since Cody was one of those Velcro dogs that did not ever want to leave my side, and since I spent a good amount of time indoors, I knew I had to do something to clean up the indoor air quality.

According to the Environmental Protection Agency (EPA), poor indoor air quality is among the top five environmental risks to public health,[vi] with levels of air pollution inside buildings two to five (and as much as one hundred) times higher than outdoor levels.[vii] And with the people of industrialized nations spending more than 90 percent of their time indoors,[viii] it should come as no surprise that many of our dogs are spending the majority of their lives indoors breathing in the same dirty indoor air that we are.

Why do buildings have such bad air quality? Many building materials such as paints, varnishes, lacquers, and cleaning and disinfecting compounds emit volatile organic chemicals into the air. The glues used in engineered wood, carpet backing, and to install flooring emit formaldehyde. And then, to top it off, we close our windows to keep in the heat during the winter and to keep in the cool air conditioning in the summer. In other words, we seal ourselves and our dogs in with pollutants that can't escape unless we let them out.

In humans, poor indoor air quality can aggravate the following conditions:

- Asthma

- Allergic reactions

- Bronchitis

- Ear and upper respiratory infections in children

I can only imagine that they cause similar issues in dogs. They just can't tell us exactly what it does. And what is poor air quality doing to your dog fighting cancer?

If you ever go to a state-of-the-art oncology ward in a human hospital, you will likely notice that the air is so very clean. There is a reason for that. Their patients are sick. Their immune systems are compromised and any complication such as poor air quality can be deadly. The same is true for your dog fighting cancer. If you can't get your dog outdoors for some good old fresh air or if the outdoor air quality is poor, then cleaning up their indoor air is critical.

One of the easiest things you can do is open up the windows. Let that fresh air in. If the weather does not permit it or if the outdoor air quality is bad, you have to do what you can to clean up the indoor air.

I also installed an air filter (which only cost around ten dollars) in the central heater during the cold months when the windows were closed, so we were at least getting cleaner air, and I would change it every month.

In addition, since my house was built in 1938 and likely had lead paint, I would wash the windowsills often with water. This was especially important in my case since the big picture window in the living room was Cody's favorite spot.

I also used a vacuum with a HEPA (High Efficiency Particulate Air) filter to vacuum the baseboards as a broom or carpet sweeper will not remove lead dust. In addition, I used a portable, high-powered HEPA air filter. Since it was expensive, I would place it in the downstairs office during the day, and bring it upstairs in the evening, where Cody and I would end our day.

I took every precaution I could to ensure that the air that Cody breathed was as clean as possible.

33 Make Pilling Your Dog Enjoyable

Aimee Quemuel

The last thing I wanted was for Cody not to trust me. I knew that I had to figure out a way to make his daily pill popping an enjoyable session.

Once I decided on a protocol for Cody, which consisted of plenty of supplements and a few Western medications, I had another challenge ahead of me: how the heck was I going to get him to take all those pills? While Cody was critically sick, his nose still worked quite well. And when I tried putting the pills in his food, he snubbed it at the first sign of a foreign substance. To him, if it was not meat or vegetables, he was not going to eat it.

I first tried pilling him by essentially shoving dozens of pills down his throat. This was not only time consuming, but stressful for Cody. He started avoiding me in fear that each time he saw me I would pry his mouth open and forcefully shove unwanted substances down his throat. The thought of Cody being upset with me, especially during this time, just broke my heart. The last thing I wanted was for Cody not to trust me. I knew that I had to figure out a way to make his daily pill popping an enjoyable session.

I also tried mixing the pills directly into Cody's food and masking the smell of the pills with fish oil, the stinkier the better. It worked initially, but Cody was on so many pills that he was bound to discover my little trick. And, sure enough, after just a few days, Cody bit into a pill. He immediately walked away from his food and seemingly threw a fit in the corner.

I then tried making meatballs. Dozens of them. I felt like that episode of Seinfeld where Newman and Kramer were making tons of sausage in Jerry's apartment. And I reeked of meat, which for a dog was heaven, but for a human, not so much. I religiously got up early every morning and started rolling meatballs. I cooked them slightly to enhance the smell. I would then proceed to shove his plethora of supplements into dozens of meatball. At first, Cody would happily eat these, but after about a month, he bit into a meatball and a supplement exploded in his mouth. If you have ever had this happen to you, you would know just how unpleasant this is, and I don't blame him for being upset. From that day forward, he refused to eat meatballs for, once again, he knew he was being tricked.

I then heard about something called Greenies® Pill Pockets®, found at http://www.greenies.com/en_US/Products/. These treats are designed to carry your dog's pill medication inside. Cody loved them. The bacon-like smell was so enticing to him that he would swallow them whole, avoiding the possibility of another exploding supplement in his mouth. However, the downside is that they are expensive and do contain sugars and some other chemicals that may not support your cancer fight, so you have to weigh the benefits of getting the pills in your dog with the fact the he/she would be getting some sugars, which could feed the cancer. Cody was taking over a dozen pills a day, and if I used them according to the instructions, it would cost nearly $150 a month. So I would put the pills in his food that I knew he would not reject and I would shove as many of the pills in each pocket that would fit. Sometimes I would even just smear a thin layer of the stuff on the pill and that was enough to get Cody to swallow them whole. This approach saved me thousands of dollars over the course of his treatment and minimized the sugars he was getting. And Cody thoroughly enjoyed them. He thought he was getting special treats. Finally, after months of trying various methods, I was able to get those important pills into Cody's system without all the stress.

Other methods include cheese balls and peanut butter (although these again would contain sugars). You can also get most supplements in liquid format and syringe them in.

Eliminate Vaccinations

Laurie Kaplan

Once a dog is diagnosed with cancer, vaccines are contraindicated and dangerous.

Laurie Kaplan, author of the best-selling book Help Your Dog Fight Cancer, *recommends that all vaccinations be diligently avoided for a dog with cancer for the remainder of that dog's life. Laurie's dog Bullet was diagnosed with lymphoma and lived for four-plus years past his diagnosis. He never received another vaccination in his last four years and four months.*

Vaccines are a medical miracle. The development of vaccinations has been singularly responsible for controlling or eradicating many diseases over the years. They can prevent acute and deadly diseases such as parvo, distemper, and rabies. However, adverse effects can result from the vaccinations themselves, and/or the manner and frequency in which they are administered, and/or the adjuvants that are added to the vaccine. According to research and volumes of anecdotal studies, vaccinations can be correlated with damage to the very immune system they are meant to protect. Research shows that vaccines may actually cause cancer.

There are about eighteen diseases your dog can be vaccinated against. Some veterinarians are overly generous in their vaccination recommendations, and will inoculate your dog against a disease that is not even a threat in your area. Some of the biggest culprits in over-vaccination are the combination vaccines such as the "5 in 1," which essentially gives a puppy or dog several different immune system challenges all at once. Increasingly, veterinarians are now recommending that each vaccination be given separately and spaced out accordingly.

Historically, veterinary practitioners have recommended annual vaccinations. However, it has been clearly established during the past decade that vaccinations are very often protective for longer than the one year suggested by vaccine manufacturers. Further, most adult dogs have adequate immunity if they have been vaccinated within the past three years. Distemper, parvo, and rabies vaccinations are all thought to provide long-lived immunity.

Every dog should be evaluated as an individual based on his risk, potential exposure to disease, and general health. Once a dog is diagnosed with cancer, however, vaccines are contraindicated and dangerous. In 'Natural Health for Dogs and Cats,' Dr. Richard Pitcairn warns that, "giving a vaccine to an animal with cancer is like pouring gasoline on a fire."[ix] Many veterinarians agree with Dr. Pitcairn's sentiments and do not recommend vaccinations for a pet with cancer.

Vaccinations required by state law, such as the rabies vaccine, may be waived. I submitted a vaccination waiver form signed by Bullet's veterinarian to NY State in 2000 and the state waived the requirement. You can print the waiver form at http://www.helpyourdogfightcancer.com/VaccineWaiver.shtml.

Once Bullet was diagnosed with cancer, he was never given another vaccination. Knowing that vaccinations often wreak havoc on the immune system, I simply did not want to take a chance.

If your dog has cancer, or has had cancer, please avoid vaccinating! If your state will not waive the requirement or if a particular fatal disease is prevalent in your area and you feel a need to provide protection against it, ask your veterinarian to titer test rather than vaccinating. Antibody titer tests indicate how strong your dog's immunity is against a certain disease, so that you can provide the vaccine only if your dog's immunity is depleted. Titer tests provide dog owners with peace of mind that their animal is protected, without over vaccinating.

Use Nontoxic Lawn and Garden Products

Laurie Kaplan

Lawn care products, including fertilizers, weed killers (herbicides), and pesticides, are the number one cause of lymphoma in dogs.

Most manufacturers of lawn care products recommend that we keep our pets off of the lawn for twenty-four hours after application, but this is not an adequate precaution. Lawn care products, including fertilizers, weed killers (herbicides), and pesticides, are the number one cause of lymphoma in dogs. According to a recent Examiner.com article, "Dogs exposed to herbicide-treated lawns and gardens can double their chance of developing canine lymphoma."[x]

I don't feel that my health is in danger from lawn care chemicals—then again, it's been many years since I gave up rolling around on my front lawn or digging in the dirt. I don't eat grass laden with chemicals and I don't lick the bottoms of my shoes or feet when I come inside. I'm guessing that you don't do these things either, but Bullet did and, most likely, your dog does too. These chemicals are *not* safe for our dogs because dogs can't help but inhale the powders, with their noses just inches from the ground, and lick pools of water that have accumulated, invisibly laced with nasty toxins.

What can you do to protect your dog from carcinogens in lawn care products? Find natural, organic, nontoxic lawn care products. Your local garden center can help you choose one, or you can research on the Internet to find the one that fits your needs. A garden/weed flamer, which uses propane-fueled heat, can be used to kill weeds safely without the use of any chemicals.

You can also pour boiling water on small clumps of unwanted growth. Vinegar kills weeds too, but it also kills grass, so use vinegar only on the rogue weeds on your driveway or walkway.

If you live in a condo or an apartment, ask the management company if the landscaping products they use contain pesticides or herbicides. If so, ask them to post flags after each treatment is applied and remember to keep your dog off the grass for a week after each treatment. Canvas your neighbors and compile a petition signed by all residents who want safe products used on the property. Submit the petition to the management. There is strength in numbers, and this will validate and strengthen your position. The petition will be more persuasive and effective if it includes a statement saying that signers are willing to bear a nominal increase in monthly management or commons fees during the summer months to account for the higher price of natural products.

Now that your property is safe, what about the products your neighbors use on their lawns? Powders are easily blown from one property to another or carried by wild critters, human visitors, or delivery people and carried right onto your pristine yard, despite all of your precautions! Keep a container of hand-sanitizer wipes by the door and wipe your dog's paws before he enters to remove pesticide residue. As for the indoors, I recommend a "no shoes in the house" rule. Keep your floors and carpets clean and free of chemical deposits from the shoes of visitors. Your pets will be safe from those chemicals, and when you stretch out on the floor to read a book or watch your favorite TV show, you won't be laying in a bed of toxins.

36 Use Nontoxic Organic Cleaners

Rosemary Levesque

Rosemary Levesque focused on removing toxins as her primary cancer-fighting tool. Her dog Ginger defied the hemangiosarcoma odds and lived sixteen months post-diagnosis.

Dog cancers are increasing at the same rate as human cancers, causing researchers to look more closely at a shared environmental pathogenesis.

According to the Environmental Working Group April 2008 report, "Dogs and cats were contaminated with 48 of 70 industrial chemicals tested, including 43 chemicals at levels higher than those typically found in people."[xi]

While humans are vulnerable to the effects of perpetual exposure to chemicals, including those in common household products, dogs are at even greater risk due to their faster metabolisms, smaller body sizes, and direct contact with the floor and furniture where most toxins are found. If your dog is currently fighting cancer, exposing him or her to additional carcinogens will certainly not bode well for his fight. So the bottom line is: don't use chemical-based cleaners.

My personal rule of thumb for any product I purchase, including household cleaners, is simply this: if you can't conceivably consume the ingredients, don't use it. Another telling sign of the true danger that lurks within is a warning label that says, "Keep off of skin." This is just another way of saying the product is toxic.

Let's take a look at a few examples of just how toxic household cleaners can be:

- Formaldehyde, a key ingredient in most floor cleaners, is an irritant that affects the skin, eyes, and throats of pets and humans and has been classified as a known human carcinogen (cancer-causing substance) by the International Agency for Research on Cancer and as a probable human carcinogen by the U.S. Environmental Protection Agency.[xii]

- Perchloroethylene (also known as PERC), another chemical found in floor cleaners and often used by dry cleaners, affects the central nervous system and has been shown to cause cancer in animals. Dogs may experience loss of appetite, nausea, tremors or dizziness after ingesting perchloroethylene. Laboratory studies show that PERC causes kidney and liver damage and cancer in animals exposed repeatedly by inhalation and by mouth.[xiii]

- Alkylphenols, the chemicals that produce the suds in many household cleaning products, have been linked to breast cancer.[xiv] Unspayed dogs develop mammary tumors at four times the rate that women do, putting them at even greater risk cancer.[xv]

This is just a very small sampling of chemicals that we unknowingly expose our dogs to everyday—from floor cleaners to laundry detergents and fabric softeners, to scented candles and deodorizers. All you have to do is read the label. Pick an ingredient and do a Google search on it and chances are it is linked to some adverse health effect, including cancer.

Even before Ginger was diagnosed, we used water and vinegar to clean just about everything. A bucket of hot water containing a cup of white vinegar will clean, disinfect, and deodorize without creating a health hazard to pets and humans. You do not have to rinse this nontoxic solution. The vinegar smell disappears when the solution dries, leaving the surface fresh and clean.

There is no reason to expose ourselves and our pets, especially our dogs fighting cancer, to toxic household cleaners when there are now many affordable lines of organic cleaning products available at most grocery stores. In addition, there are countless books and articles on making one's own effective household cleaners for far less than the cost of conventional cleaning products. A few resources can be found at:

- http://www.carthcasy.com/live_nontoxic_solutions.htm
- http://altmedicine.about.com/cs/allergiesasthma/a/HouseholdClean.htm
- http://www.doityourself.com/stry/cleaners

37 Use Natural Flea and Tick Remedies

Aimee Quemuel

In a healthy dog, the effects of flea and tick pesticides are not immediately apparent, however, in a dog fighting cancer, they could be deadly.

Frontline, Advantage, flea collars, and other traditional flea remedies are nothing but low-grade poisons. In a healthy dog, the effects of flea and tick pesticides are not immediately apparent (though one could argue that they are slowly decreasing your dog's immunity); however, in a dog fighting cancer, they could be deadly.

For years, I used Frontline on Cody. Once he got the cancer diagnosis, one of my conventional veterinarians told me I should stop using it immediately. Why? Because it is a pesticide, she said. So, essentially, one of the tools I thought was keeping him in good health and recommended by my conventional veterinarian was likely a contributor to his current condition.

So what do you do? Fleas and ticks are unpleasant. They are not only stressful to your dog and your family, they can also cause a handful of diseases—something your dog with cancer does not need.

With just a little digging, I quickly discovered that there are plenty of natural alternatives that kill the fleas and are safe for your dog. Lemon, lavender, peppermint, cedar, lemongrass, and citronella repel fleas, and rose geranium and cedar are good for repelling ticks.

To prevent fleas and ticks, in addition to a healthy raw diet, during flea season, I sprayed Cody every few days with a natural spray made of cedar and rosemary. Originally I used NaturVet®'s herbal flea spray, but then started making my own to keep costs down. The recipe is listed in Appendix E.

I was fortunate enough to not live in a tick-infested area. I know they are tougher to deal with than fleas. If I did live in such an area, I would double up on the oils especially effective at repelling ticks: cedar wood and rose geranium.

Just in case Cody had a flea or two that I was not aware of, I also soaked him weekly with just plain old water, or I let him go swimming, which was one of his favorite things to do anyways. Fleas drown and to kill them just requires water, but you have to make sure your dog is completely soaked. No flea shampoo required.

In addition, I would vacuum the floors daily and wash Cody's bedding weekly. This ensured that if a flea or two did make it into the house, I broke the reproduction cycle. In the areas where I had carpet, I used regular table salt as a natural flea carpet powder. I would sprinkle, let it sit for a few days, and then vacuum. This does not kill adult fleas, but it prevents flea eggs from hatching by dehydrating them.

From the moment I heard the cancer word, I used all natural remedies on Cody and as far as I know, he never got a single flea again—even through an entire summer at the beach in Ventura, California. As a side note, the dog who lived downstairs and Cody often played with had a horrible bout with fleas, despite being on Frontline. He is likely the one that caused a minor flea infestation in the house, but they never bit Cody or my other dog CJ; they went after my nephew and me. In retrospect, I should have sprayed the flea spray on my nephew and myself. Why not? It is completely safe.

38 Use Nontoxic Toys and Bedding

Aimee Quemuel and Natalie Stemp

There is no regulation governing the toxicity of dog toys resulting in toxic levels of lead, chromium, arsenic, and mercury in many pet toys sold in the United States.

Carcinogens and toxins are everywhere. Every day it seems that we learn of yet another carcinogen in our home. At this point, you are likely acutely aware of why toxins are so bad for your dog fighting cancer. Carcinogens are substances that cause cancer. So if your dog is currently fighting cancer, you don't want to surround them with the very substances that might have allowed the cancer cells to grow out of control in the first place.

Don't be fooled by the cute packaging. Toys that you get for your dog can be loaded with dangerous toxins. There is no regulation governing the toxicity of dog toys resulting in toxic levels of lead, chromium, arsenic, and mercury in many pet toys sold in the United States. Dogs don't have hands, so they carry their toys in their mouths, transferring these harmful toxins straight into their systems.

A press release put out by the American Veterinary Medical Association (AVMA) stated that "they were concerned about recent reports of lead contamination in toys."[xvi]

Here is an excerpt from the release:

Independent tests by Trace Laboratories, Inc. in Illinois and ExperTox Analytical Laboratories in Texas found the presence of lead and other toxic chemicals on randomly selected toys purchased in American stores. The highest level of lead found was 30,000 parts per million (ppm) in the paint on a pet toy. The Consumer Product Safety

Commission (CPSC) enforces a federal standard for lead in paint intended for children's products, which is 600 ppm, according to CPSC spokesperson Ed Kang, but there is no federal standard for lead in pet toys.

Dr. Frederick Oehme, professor of toxicology and diagnostic medicine at Kansas State University, said symptoms of lead poisoning are vague in pets but can include a slightly anorexic appearance and a slight loss of appetite, slight behavior changes that include twitching, and whining while sleeping. In more advanced cases of lead poisoning, there are neurological symptoms that include mild to severe seizures. Dr. Oehme said if symptoms are present in your pet, consult your veterinarian for a diagnosis.

And what about the beds they sleep on, many of which are drenched in flame retardants? According to Wikipedia, chemicals in flame retardants are "considered harmful, having been linked to liver, thyroid, reproductive/developmental and neurological effects."[xvii] Even the beds that don't use flame retardants can contain toxic dyes. Your safest bet is to buy an organic bed.

Natalie Stemp recommends that you:

- Look for toys made of nontoxic materials and azo-free dyes.

- Do not buy toys your dog can easily ingest. Even nontoxic things are not meant to be ingested, and you don't want to add yet another bout of illness for your dog.

- If your dog is an avid chewer, don't get toys your dog can easily tear or break off pieces.

- If possible, monitor all toy-play sessions.

Why risk it? The solution is simple. Buy nontoxic toys and bedding. There are many options available now. You just need to do a little more due diligence.

39 Monitor Progress

Ilene Powell

When battling canine cancer, you should not fight blindly and should try to stay ahead of it.

Using an integrative approach, Labrador Retriever Mali survived hemangiosarcoma more than four years. Diagnosed at seven years old, Mali's owner, Ilene Powell, says that regular checkups were critical in fine-tuning Mali's treatment plan and were key in her incredible journey of survival.

Even after Mali survived past her original prognosis of nine to fifteen months with chemo or a few months without treatment, regular checkups were a critical part of her treatment plan. Without blood tests and ultrasounds, we would not have been able to fine-tune our approach. In other words, our treatment plan could have been a shot in the dark.

Especially if you are using traditional medicines and/or supplements as part of your treatment plan, it is important to ensure that the medicines and supplements are still doing their job and are not interfering with your dog's overall health. A dog's system can become accustomed to supplements, so you might have to "pulse" supplement use. This can mean giving them for a period of time, taking them off, and then repeating the use. Regular blood tests can give you granular insight into whether or not the medicines and supplements you are using are still working and not causing harm.

At the beginning of Mali's cancer battle, we did chest X-rays, ultrasounds, and a complete blood test every month. When Mali's cancer was deemed in "remission" or dormant, we reduced tests to every two to three months. The tests can get expensive, but, as Rebecca Clark points out in Rule 11, Funding Your Cancer Fight, money does not have to hinder your ability to get the best treatment possible, as there are now many organizations to help. I am forever grateful to Canine Cancer Awareness, http://caninecancerawareness.org/. Without them, I would not have been able to afford Mali's exhaustive treatment plan, including the regular tests we did to ensure our plan was still working.

One of the most invaluable tests we used for Mali was a complete blood count (CBC). A CBC is one of the most commonly ordered blood tests and calculates the cellular elements of your dog's blood. These calculations are generally determined by special machines that analyze the different components of blood in less than a minute. The test is performed by obtaining a few milliliters (one to two teaspoons) of blood from your dog. A simple procedure, yet the results rendered are invaluable. Here are some examples of how you might use results from a blood test:

- The test can determine if your dog is anemic.

- The test can also tell if there is a vitamin B12 deficiency.

- The test can determine low platelet counts, which, in Mali's cancer, could likely be a result of a bleeding tumor, one of the characteristics of hemangiosarcoma.

- The test can monitor organ function, which can tell you how your dog is handling the medicines, supplements, and/or diet.

This is just a sample of some of the results a blood test would reveal. However, you simply would not be armed with this information without a blood test.

Another useful and safe test is the ultrasound. The most well-known application of ultrasound is its use in sonography to produce pictures of fetuses in the human womb. The ultrasound could determine even the slightest changes in your dog's internal organs and could reveal the very beginnings of a tumor. Again, this insight could help you determine your next maneuver in your dog's cancer fight.

When battling canine cancer, you should not fight blindly and should try to stay ahead of it. Monitoring organ health and function and addressing issues such as anemia, vitamin B12 deficiencies, and low platelet count could mitigate future complications and could mean all the difference in the world in your dog's cancer fight.

40 Be Mindful of Other Diseases

Aimee Quemuel

If you should be so lucky to beat out cancer, remember that just because you defeated cancer doesn't mean you are immune to other diseases and mishaps.

During a cancer battle, many dog owners tend to focus so intensely on the cancer that they forget that there are plenty of other diseases that can end their dogs lives prematurely. I learned firsthand the importance of being mindful of other diseases and mishaps.

Cody's initial prognosis was so grave that the veterinarians gave him just a few days to live. Yet, after five months of fighting what veterinarians called an incurable cancer, Cody's tumors on his liver and heart disappeared without chemo and without surgery. This was not a case of living with cancer longer than expected. It was a case of *reversed cancer*. It was amazing to watch. With the tumors in his liver and heart gone, Cody was now a candidate for surgery to remove his spleen, the only remaining tumor.

Cody's surgery went over without a hitch and he was officially in remission. I was ecstatic. I was on top of the world. I felt like I had won the greatest battle of my life. We defeated the cancer beast. All that hard work paid off. While I bathed in my glory, I forgot one very important detail—although his energy level was quite exuberant, better than I could remember in the past five or so years—Cody was still a twelve-year-old dog, roughly eighty-four in human years. He was not that spry, fluffy puppy I remember receiving as a Christmas gift so many years ago.

In Rule 16, Let Your Dog Live Life to the Fullest, Lisa Alford and Pamela Storto touched upon letting your dog live life to the fullest, while keeping in mind that there are limits. To that end, let me tell you firsthand just how important that is.

At twelve years old, I was letting Cody jump in and out of my SUV, which was about three feet off the ground. This was pretty much a daily occurrence since Cody went with me everywhere. I had a ramp, but it was so cumbersome to use. I got a little lazy. To be honest, I think I felt a little invincible, like there was nothing we couldn't defeat. After all, we had done the impossible. But, as the saying goes, all good things must come to an end. And boy did they.

When you live at the beach, the wind is not your friend. The wind had been particularly cruel, creating massive sand piles throughout my driveway, the snow equivalent of ice patches. In other words, it was very slippery. And one day, Cody jumped out of the car and slipped onto his back. He popped right back up so I assumed all was fine. Within a few days, he started walking funny. Like nothing I had ever witnessed, a swagger of sorts. But I still continued on with our walks. He still walked up and down a huge flight of stairs to my upstairs condo. Less than a week later, he was completely paralyzed in the hind legs.

While I tried for another miracle, even going so far as to get him a wheelchair, the paralysis was the beginning of the end. I never did the tests to determine what exactly went wrong—whether it was a spinal injury due to the fall or perhaps a new tumor pressed against his spine, but my gut tells me it was avoidable. Let me be clear. This is not about blame. I know I did the best I could for Cody. But this book is all about lessons learned. And if you should be so lucky to beat out cancer, remember that just because you defeated cancer doesn't mean you are immune to other diseases and mishaps.

41

Know When to Let Go

Aimee Quemuel and Laurie Kaplan

During a battle against cancer, we may anticipate that the loss will come soon, but knowing this in our heads does not make us "ready" in our hearts.

Losing a beloved pet is never easy, whether death comes early from a dreaded disease such as cancer or at a ripe old age from natural causes. During a battle against cancer, we may anticipate that the loss will come soon, but knowing this in our heads does not make us "ready" in our hearts. If a dog survives cancer, there is no doubt that the loss will come someday, no matter what.

We all hope that our pups will have the great fortune to go to the fabled Rainbow Bridge at a ripe old age, naturally and at home in our arms. More often, however, we have to participate in the decision to help them start that journey. This is an unspeakably painful decision to make, but at the same time it is a gift that we are empowered to give our dogs, to release them from pain and suffering. It is a gift that requires great emotional strength, and the willingness to take on the pain of loss ourselves rather than watch our pups go through more pain.

When is it time to stop fighting cancer? This is a very personal decision. Laurie Kaplan, author of *Help Your Dog Fight Cancer* and fellow dog cancer fighter, offers a few tips to help you make this decision with clarity and confidence:

- When treatment is not effective and there are no other treatment options with any promise of success.

- When your dog is suffering "too much" from the effects of the disease or the treatment. (This is a judgment call that only you can make. You are the only one who can evaluate your dog's quality of life, his level of suffering, and his ability to continue to battle.)
- When you determine that it's time to stop fighting because you, your family, or your dog can no longer fight.

Once you make your decision, do everything you can to make your dog as comfortable as possible. If your dog is in extreme pain, you will know it is time. The day I released Cody, he was wincing from the pain of internal bleeding. The look in his eyes told me he was tired of fighting. I knew releasing him from his pain was the last act of kindness that I could show my beloved dog. Just before the veterinarian administered the euthanizing drug, Cody lifted his head and looked me in the eyes thanking me for all I had done. It was the saddest day of my life, yet at the same time the most inspirational, as it has changed me for the better in so many ways. Laurie Kaplan beautifully describes euthanasia as "the ultimate sacrifice because, at this point, their suffering ends and ours begins."

After your dog is gone, it is normal to feel a deep sense of loss. There are an increasing number of support groups and outlets for grieving pet owners (see Appendix F for a list of resources for pet loss). The bond you had with your dog was real. And those that have ever experienced that special relationship with a dog will understand. Just like the decision to let your dog go or to stop treatment is a personal choice, so is the way you grieve. I am certainly not an expert on grieving, but I do know that losing Cody was unlike any other pain I have ever felt. It has been nearly over two years since I released Cody, and I still miss him each and every day. At times I feel like something might be wrong with me, as the pain is still quite sharp. It seems that the deeper you love, the harder it is to let go. If I had the choice, would I do it all again? Absolutely. And that is the "thing" that keeps me going, the reason I will always be a dog owner. The beauty these amazing creatures called dogs bring into your life is, frankly, what life is all about.

42

These Are Our Rules. What Are Yours?

Aimee Quemuel

Tell us your story at FightDogCancer.com and you will be contributing to something that will be used to save dogs for years to come. Together, with our collective knowledge, we can save our dogs.

When I first decided to write this book, I envisioned telling my own personal journey with dog cancer. A tale that would describe just how special Cody was and why losing him was like losing a piece of my soul. It would talk about how we fought and defeated the cancer beast, why my approach worked, and why others should consider using my method for attacking cancer. But then I realized that I was not alone in this journey, that there were thousands of people, perhaps even millions, in the same boat as I was, people that were or are just as connected to their dogs as I was to Cody, and, perhaps, they were also dog cancer survivors in one form or another.

I then sat down to try to recall the moments during the battle that I felt lost. I remembered how difficult it was to find tales of survival and how very sad that made me. I also remembered how I felt when I did find those stories of survival. It was like the light was turned on, an immense feeling of hope that perhaps my Cody could be one of those miracle dogs. The more I thought about it, the more it was clear that this book needed go beyond a tale of a girl and her dog. It needed to be a collective book of knowledge from dog owners all over the country that not only talked about their tales of survival, but also the deep connection they shared with their dogs. After all, much of my treatment plan for Cody was the result of the knowledge of past dog cancer warriors. As so it began—a journey to create a book of inspiration filled with bits of knowledge from dog cancer survivors.

While I still believe there are definite rules that make sense for all cancers—like removing all possible toxins from your dog's environment and feeding a cancer-fighting diet—this book has taught me that there are many ways to skin a cat (so to speak, and no offense to cat lovers). Each dog owner I interviewed approached their cancer journey slightly differently. There were a plethora of methods used-traditional, holistic, or just plain old love and attention. But they all had a survival story. *Their dogs all survived cancer anywhere from a year to six and a half years; translated into human years, that is quite significant.*

Initially, I thought finding stories of survival would be difficult. A little digging proved me wrong. I literally made a few phone calls and posted to a couple of dog-related groups, and the stories came pouring in. I discovered that 1 out of 3 dogs will have cancer in their lives.[xviii] With 77.5 million dogs in the U.S. alone, that means there are roughly 25.8 million dogs with cancer; each with a story to tell and each with a bit of wisdom that we can all learn from. The twenty-two contributors to this book are just a small sampling of the knowledge out there.

Imagine what we could do if we were able to cull our collective knowledge in one place. Beyond this book, I have started a new Web site called FightDogCancer.com (see Appendix G) with that exact goal in mind: to gather as many dog cancer stories as possible in one place so that those currently in battle can learn from our collective wisdom.

These are our rules. What are yours? Tell us your story at http://www.fightdogcancer.com and you will be contributing to something that will be used to save dogs for years to come. Together, with our collective knowledge, we can save our dogs.

100 percent of the author's proceeds will be donated to dog cancer nonprofits.

A Contributors' Biographies

Elizabeth Heller and Osquer

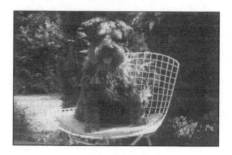

Owner's name: Elizabeth Heller
Where they live: Lexington, Massachusetts
Dog's name: Osquer
Dog's breed: Miniature Schnauzer
Age at diagnosis: 12 years
Prognosis: 6 months to a year
Outcome: 3 years
Primary treatment: Shark cartilage
Email: rellehe1@aol.com

After a divorce, Elizabeth Heller became the sole caregiver of Osquer, a loving, sweet Miniature Schnauzer, who quickly became more than just a dog. He was family. Elizabeth's son used to jokingly call him "her husband." What a friend Osquer became to Elizabeth. They went everywhere together. Even to the end, Elizabeth used to walk him in a stroller. At twelve years old, Osquer was diagnosed with cancer and given a year to live at most. Elizabeth credits a shark cartilage regimen for three more quality years of life with her beloved Miniature Schnauzer, Osquer.

Caryn Wilson and Beanny

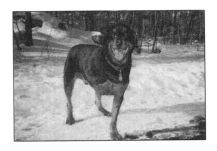

Owner's name: Caryn Wilson
Where they live: Andover, Massachusetts
Dog's name: Beanny
Dog's breed: Rottweiler
Type of cancer: Osteosarcoma
Age at diagnosis: 6½ years
Prognosis: 6 months to a year
Outcome: 21 months
Primary treatment: Surgery, chemotherapy, supplements, and herbs
Email: director@caninecancer.com
Web address: http://www.caninecancer.com

Caryn Wilson's first personal experience with cancer was with her dog named Puma, who also had osteosarcoma. That was fourteen years ago. Since then, Caryn has had two other dogs with osteosarcoma.

When her second dog, Beanny, was diagnosed and given about a year to live, she began to read every book, every medical journal, every Internet site, and every clinical trial she could find. She explored conventional therapies and alternative and holistic treatments. Nothing was too outlandish to try. She wanted desperately to cure him, or at least give him longer to live than Puma had (he died six months after diagnosis). During her research process, Caryn read of an herbal remedy called Essiac tea. Beanny lived twenty-one months post his diagnosis and Caryn credits the Essiac tea. Compelled to help others fighting dog cancer, in February 2007, Caryn launched CanineCancer.com, an informational site on dog cancer.

Sherri Cooper and Asia

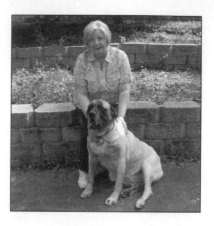

Owner's name: Sherri Cooper
Where they live: Okemos, Michigan
Dog's name: Asia
Dog's breed: English Mastiff
Type of cancer: Stomach cancer
Age at diagnosis: 8 years
Prognosis: 1–3 months
Outcome: 2 years and 3 months to date
Primary treatment: Steroids
Email: scooper1jonus@sbcglobal.net

In February 2008, Sherri Cooper's English Mastiff, who normally had a veracious appetite, quit eating altogether, so Sherri immediately took her to the veterinarian. An ultrasound revealed a softball-sized tumor in her stomach. A biopsy determined it was malignant. With such a grim prognosis, Sherri considered euthanizing, but decided to at least give Asia a chance to fight. Asia was immediately put on steroids. The next week, Sherri brought her in for a checkup. The very palpable tumor could not be found. So the veterinarian did another ultrasound and miraculously the tumor was gone.

Sherri kept Asia on steroids for another couple of months, but had to stop as steroids stimulate the appetite and Asia started eating everything in sight, including all of her toys. That was exactly one year ago, and she is still doing fine and cancer-free. Sherri also credits lots of prayers to Asia's recovery.

Jeanne Arsenault and Bailey

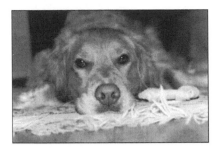

Owner's name: Jeanne Arsenault
Where they live: Saugus, Massachusetts
Dog's name: Bailey
Dog's breed: Golden Retriever/Cocker Spaniel mix
Type of cancer: Prostate
Age at diagnosis: 10½ years
Prognosis: 3–4 months with no treatment, 10 months with chemo
Outcome: 21 months
Primary treatment: Healing sessions, diet, and herbs
Email/Web address: jmarsenault@comcast.net

At ten and a half years old, Jeanne Arsenault's Golden Retriever/Cocker Spaniel mix, Bailey, was diagnosed with prostate cancer and given three to four months to live with no treatment, and ten months with chemo. With the help of Rolando Masse of Healing Hands, http://www.rolandoshealinghands.com, Jeanne learned how to give Bailey Reiki, a Japanese technique for stress reduction and relaxation. Bailey survived twenty-one months after his initial diagnosis, with no conventional treatment, and died of natural causes. A completely natural approach that included healing sessions, a natural diet, and herbs was used in this success story. No chemo or surgery.

No other person, not one thing
Has ever left me with quite this much sting.
You were my child, my companion
A true loyal friend
And you will live on in my heart
Until we meet again.

Rest peacefully now Bailey and know your Momma loves you.

Lynn Browne and Samson

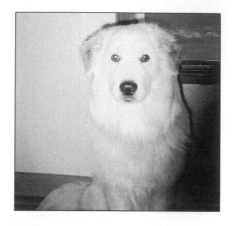

Owner's name: Lynn Browne
Where they live: Greenfield Center, New York
Dog's name: Samson
Dog's breed: Great Pyrenees
Type of cancer: Hemangiosarcoma in the spleen
Age at diagnosis: 13 years
Prognosis: 3 months with surgery and if it did not spread
Outcome: As of October 2009, 17 months
Primary treatment: Surgery, Chinese herbs, and chiropractic adjustments

At thriteen years old, Samson, a Great Pyrenees, was diagnosed with incurable hemangiosarcoma of the spleen and given three months to live, even with surgery. Using a combination of Western and Eastern approaches, Samson is living out his senior years in Greenfield Center, New York, with his owner Lynn Browne. At the time of this writing, Samson has survived seventeen cancer-free months.

Rebecca Clark, Kibo and Sana

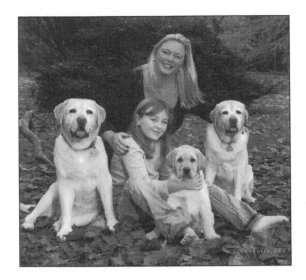

Owner's name: Rebecca Clark
Where they live: Newport, Rhode Island
Dogs' names: Kibo and Sana
Dogs' breed: Labrador Retrievers
Types of cancer: Mast cell tumor and lymphoma
Ages at diagnosis: Kibo, 11; Sana, 6
Prognoses: Kibo, 4–6 weeks without chemotherapy; longer with Sana
Outcomes: 3 years for Sana; 1 year, 2 months for Kibo
Email: NwptRN@yahoo.com

Rebecca Clark from Newport, Rhode Island was first affected by canine cancer in 2006, when her Yellow Lab, Sana, age six at the time, was diagnosed with mast cell cancer. He had three surgeries to remove the tumors, and the veterinarian was able to get clean margins, which gave him a good prognosis.

Then in December 2008, cancer reared its ugly head once again when Rebecca's other Yellow Lab, Kibo, was diagnosed with Lymphoma at age eleven. Overwhelmed with the expenses, Rebecca turned to her community and the Magic Bullet Fund, http://www.themagicbulletfund.org, to get Kibo the necessary care. After 14 months, in February 2010, Kibo lost his battle to cancer. Rebecca also lost Sana in June of 2009, due to a mast cell cancer recurrence.

Suzanne Morrone and Zara

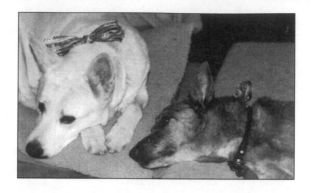

Owner's name: Suzanne Morrone
Where they live: San Jose, California
Dog's name: Zara
Dog's breed: Pitt Bull/Wolf Mix
Type of cancer: Mast cell tumor hind left/right legs
Age at diagnosis: 7 years
Prognosis: Poor without further treatment
Outcome: 6 years
Email: gowithdog@sbcglobal.net

Contrary to the stereotype of her breed, Zara, a Pitt Bull/Wolf mix, was a gentle, shy giant and mother figure to the all the animals in the house—from her seizure-prone dog-mate Hopi to several cats and even the turtles. At seven years old, she was diagnosed with mast cell cancer and given a poor prognosis without further treatment. Surgery, radiation, and lots of love were the treatments that her owner Suzanne Morrone decided on. Zara lived another six years to the ripe old age of thirteen, which, especially for a dog of her size, was a full life.

Erik Johnson and Kita

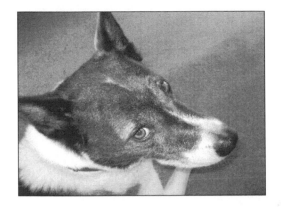

Owner's name: Erik Johnson
Where they live: Tucson, Arizona
Dog's name: Kita
Dog's breed: Akita mix
Type of cancer: Prostate and bladder cancer
Age at diagnosis: 9 years
Prognosis: 2–3 months
Outcome: 17 months
Primary treatment: Herbs
Email: erik@pet-helper.com
Web address: http://www.pet-helper.com

Erik Johnson grew up in Washington State and migrated to California where he owned and eventually sold a highly successful computer support business in Silicon Valley.

Moving to Arizona to be closer to family, Erik and his wife now operate several health-related businesses including Healthy Living Solutions, http://www.hls-herbs.com, and The Internet Health Store, http://www.theInternethealthstore.com, featuring herbal solutions and other products for people, and Healthy Pet Solutions, http://www.pet-helper.com, featuring herbals and other items for dogs, cats, and other family animals.

An active community volunteer with the Lions Club, Erik also makes time for racquetball (and driving lessons) with his teenage son and long walks with his new dog, Bella.

Laurie Kaplan and Bullet

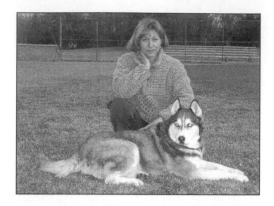

Owner's name: Laurie Kaplan
Where they live: Briarcliff, New York
Dog's name: Bullet
Dog's breed: Siberian Husky
Type of cancer: Lymphoma
Age at diagnosis: 9 years, 4 months
Prognosis: 1 month without chemo; 1 year with chemo
Outcome: 4 years and 4 months
Primary treatment: Chemo, diet and supplements, love and adoration!
Email: laurie.kaplan@themagicbulletfund.org
Web address: http://www.themagicbulletfund.org,
http://www.helpyourdogfightcancer.com

Laurie Kaplan is the author of *Help Your Dog Fight Cancer.*

As a result of her own battle with dog cancer, Laurie founded the Magic Bullet Fund. This nonprofit provides financial assistance for families that have dogs with cancer but are financially unable to provide treatment. (Apply for help or donate to help others at http://www.themagicbulletfund.org.)

Lisa Alford and Lucy

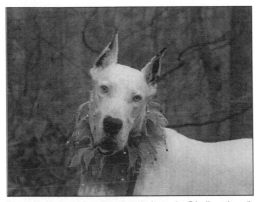

Photo by Kathryn Goodwin (katclarityworks@bellsouth.net)

Owner's name: Lisa Alford
Where they live: Asheville, North Carolina
Dog's name: Lucy
Dog's breed: Great Dane
Type of cancer: Thyroid and subcutaneous hemangiosarcoma
Age at diagnosis: 5½ years
Prognosis: 3 months to a year
Outcome: 19 months to date (still alive as of November 2009)
Primary treatment: Surgery, chemotherapy, supplements, and herbs
Email: lisa.alford@mac.com
Web address: http://www.greatdanefriends.com

An absolute sweetheart from the day she came into Lisa Alford's life, Lucy, a stunning white Great Dane, was meant to do good things with her life. With no formal training, Lucy just seemed to "get it." Calm, peaceful, and friendly, she always listens and is always well behaved.

In May 2008, at just five and a half years old, Lucy was diagnosed with two different types of cancer (subcutaneous hemangiosarcoma and thyroid) plus heart disease (cardiomyopathy). Needless to say, Lisa, her owner, was heartbroken. But Lisa decided early on that she was not going to let the cancer diagnosis spoil her time with Lucy. She was not going to let the cancer stop them from living. So, in September 2009, after chemotherapy, surgery, and nutrition therapy, Lucy became an official therapy dog visiting the pediatric floors at the local hospital and she absolutely loves it.

Lisa is a proud part of the rescue, Great Dane Friends, http://www.greatdanefriends.com), dedicated to saving Danes and other dogs, especially ones that may be passed up by other rescues due to special needs.

Pamela Storto and Sierra

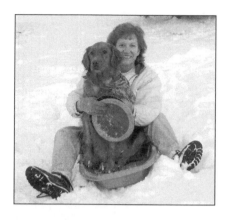

Owner's name: Pamela Storto
Where they live: Litchfield, Maine
Dog's name: Sierra
Dog's breed: Golden Retriever
Type of cancer: Lymphoma
Age at diagnosis: 3½ years
Prognosis: 4–5 weeks without chemotherapy; 4 months with chemo
Outcome: 13 wonderful months
Primary treatment: Chemotherapy
Email: lpam2527@aol.com
Web address: http://www.caninecancerawareness.org

Pamela Storto's journey with dog cancer began when her young, vibrant Sierra, a three-and-a-half-year-old Golden Retriever, was diagnosed with lymphoma. Sierra was treated with the Wisconsin Protocol (chemotherapy), and lived thirteen additional and wonderful months. So moved by the experience, Pamela quit her job to dedicate her life to fighting dog cancer. Though Sierra's life was short, her legacy lives on through Canine Cancer Awareness, a nonprofit organization started by Pamela that raises funds to care for dogs with cancer whose owners are financially unable to provide treatment. More information can be found at http://www.caninecancerawareness.org.

Jane and Alan Luba, and Oscar

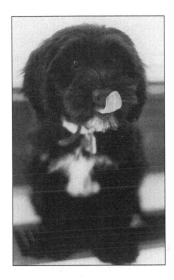

Owner's name: Jane and Alan Luba
Where they live: Centreville, Virginia
Dog's name: Oscar
Dog's breed: Cockapoo
Type of cancer: Mast cell
Age at diagnosis: 10 years
Prognosis: 3 months without treatment
Outcome: 3 years
Primary treatment: Surgery, chemotherapy, and radiation
Email: JaneLuba@Verizon.net

At ten years old, Jane Luba's dog, Oscar, also known in the Luba family as "the happiest dog on the earth," was diagnosed with mast cell cancer. Using surgery, radiation, and chemotherapy, happy-go-lucky Oscar fought two different bouts of cancer and lived three more exuberant, cancer-free years.

Kristine Tanzillo and Sheldon

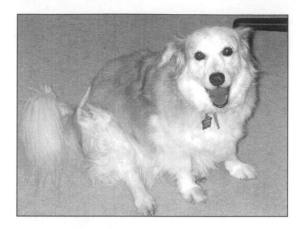

Owner's name: Kristine Tanzillo
Where they live: Canton, Texas
Dog's name: Sheldon
Dog's breed: Corgi Sheltie Mix
Type of cancer: Stomach
Age at diagnosis: 14¾ years
Prognosis: 6 weeks
Outcome: 1 year and 4 months
Primary treatment: Food
Email/Web address: kristine@duxpr.com

Kristine Tanzillo had just lost her other dog when she saw a woman was giving away puppies in a Walmart parking lot. She just couldn't resist, and that was the start of more than fourteen beautiful years with Sheldon. The small but mighty protector of the family, Sheldon was not the outwardly friendly type to anyone outside the family. Even as a puppy, he would carefully observe his environment as if to be patrolling for intruders. At nearly fifteen years old, Sheldon was diagnosed with stomach cancer and, although he lived a long life for a dog, Kristine just wanted to make sure Sheldon was as comfortable as possible. Given only six weeks to live, Sheldon miraculously made it to his sixteenth birthday without treatment beyond food.

Robin Barbosa and Disnay

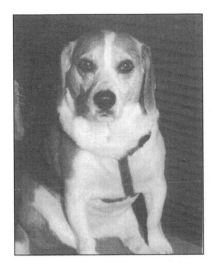

Owner's name: Robin Barbosa
Where they live: Leonia, New Jersey
Dog's name: Disnay (pronounced Disney),
Dog's breed: Beagle
Type of cancer: Mast cell tumor
Age at diagnosis: 9 years and 8 months
Prognosis: 2 years
Outcome: 6½ years to the ripe old age of 16
Primary treatment: Surgery and raw vegetable diet
Email: robspecbarb@hotmail.com

At 9 years and 8 months, Disnay (pronounced Disney) was diagnosed with mast cell cancer. Robin opted for surgery. Because the tumor was on her neck and so close to vital organs, the surgeon did not get clean margins, which gave her only two years at best. After researching, Robin discovered how bad her previous diet of kibble was for cancer. So she started making her food, which consisted of lots of finely grated raw vegetables, chicken, and flaxseed. Long story short, the diet, in addition to lots of prayer, gave Robin's precious Disnay a full, long life.

Ilene Powell and Mali

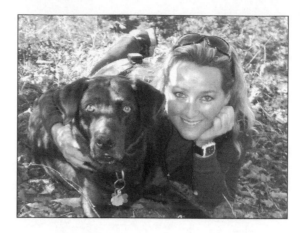

Owner's name: Ilene Powell
Where they live: New Orleans, Louisiana
Dog's name: Mali
Dog's breed: Labrador Retriever
Type of cancer: Hemangiosarcoma (spleen)
Age at diagnosis: 7½ years
Prognosis: 2–6 months without chemotherapy; 9–15 months with chemotherapy
Outcome: 4 yrs, 3 months, 2 weeks and 1 day
Primary treatment: Surgery, chemotherapy, supplements, vitamins, and herbs
Email: powellilene@yahoo.com

Known as a miracle dog in the hemangiosarcoma community, Mali survived four years post her diagnosis. Considered incurable, dogs with this type of cancer rarely reach remission and rarely live more than a few months. Using surgery, chemotherapy, supplements, vitamins, and herbs, Mali lived to see her senior years with grace and dignity. An active support group member, even after Mali passed, Ilene continues to share her incredible story of survival so that future dog cancer battles can be won.

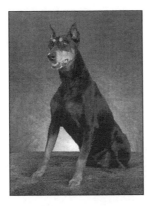

Owner's name: Jill Spencer
Where they live: West Lafayette, Indiana
Dog's name: RCi (pronounced R-C)
Dog's breed: Doberman Pinscher
Type of cancer: Fibrosarcoma (cancer of the connective tissue)
Age at diagnosis: 6 years
Prognosis: 2–3 months with no treatment; or an 80 percent chance at a possible year with radical treatment of tumor removal with four ribs, reconstruction of the ribcage, and ten weeks of radiation treatments
Outcome: 34 months with no tumor removal, no chemo, and no radiation treatments
Primary treatment: Daily exercise and a high antioxidant-supplemental immune booster containing: spirulina, chlorella, millet, flax seed, and L-glutamine
Email: jespencer@verizon.net
Web address: http://adobeangel.com/

Since childhood, dogs have been a part of Jill Spencer's life. She calls pets "fur kids," because to Jill they are family members. During her college years, she can remember feeling lost and lonely without her family dogs around. Needless to say, she has always had an innate connection with animals—a connection that has only grown stronger as the years go by.

With her own belief in the use of supplements and antioxidants to strengthen her health as well as her love for animals, it's no surprise that something happened that morphed the two great passions of Jill's life into a business aimed at helping other dogs fighting cancer and other immune system problems. A'Dobe Angel, named after Jill's beloved Doberman, RCi, who survived thirty-four months with cancer, offers the same antioxidant formula that Jill credits with RCi's miraculous story. Being able to assist other fur-kid parents dealing with serious pet health issues such as cancer, valley fever, etc., has been not only a blessing to Jill, but an opportunity to see RCi's legacy lives on—she is an angel blessing others' lives! More information about RCi and A'Dobe Angel can be found at http://adobeangel.com/.

(General disclaimer: This is our personal story. Our product is intended for animal use only. These statements have not been evaluated by the Food and Drug Administration. This product is not intended to diagnose, treat, cure, or prevent diseases. Please consult your veterinarian or pet health care professional.)

Taimi Dunn Gorman and Liwu

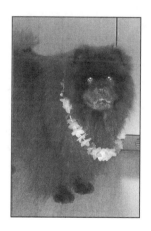

Owner's name: Taimi Dunn Gorman
Where they live: Bellingham, Washington
Dog's name: Liwu
Dog's breed: Chow Chow
Type of cancer: Liver
Age at diagnosis: 11 years
Prognosis: Weeks to months
Outcome: 18 months
Primary treatment: Mushroom supplement
Email/Web address: taimi@gormanpublicity.com

Northwest native Taimi Dunn Gorman was strictly a cat person until Chow Chow Liwu came into her life. She began taking the little black puppy to her restaurant every day, where he slept peacefully in the office and enjoyed treats each morning at the bank. His dignified, regal, and protective manner didn't hide the love he had for his family and a small, grey kitten named Alfie, who always remained his best friend.

Though Liwu was quiet and well behaved at the restaurant, there was a constant worry that the health department would find him, giving Taimi the idea of opening a restaurant for dogs next door. The Doggie Diner, later to become The Doggie Café, opened in 2000 to rave reviews and lots of press.

People Magazine, *Good Housekeeping*, and *Hello* were just a few publications enamored by the innovative concept of dogs and people dining together. Although accepted in European countries, no one had done it in the U.S. Liwu was joined by a Pug named Madeline and the two became famous, modeling doggie attire and testing the bakery's treats. The dogs and Taimi were featured on nearly every news station around the world.

Owning more than one restaurant became stressful for Taimi, who sold the famous dog cafe in 2001, wanting to visit the place with her dogs, not own it. Shortly after, she sold her "people" restaurant and became a sought-after small business consultant and publicist. Her former restaurant, The Colophon Café in Bellingham, is still as busy as ever and permits dogs at the outside tables, a nod to the famous Doggie Diner which spawned numerous imitators around the country.

Rosemary Levesque and Ginger

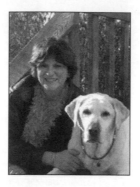

Owner's name: Rosemary Levesque and Levesque Family
Where they live: Portland, Oregon
Dog's name: Ginger
Dog's breed: Yellow Lab
Age at diagnosis: 12½ years
Prognosis: 16 days, possibly 60, if lucky
Outcome: 16 months
Primary treatment: Detoxification with Natural Cellular Defense and surgery
Email: rosemary@rosemaryssolutions.com
Web address: http://www.rosemaryssolutions.com

Rosemary is a Reiki Master, a Biologist, and an Independent Wellness Consultant with Waiora, specializing in highly effective detoxification and natural nutritional supplements. She is devoted to providing alternative and complementary health solutions for people and animals. She addresses health crises, environmental toxicity, and education for the prevention of disease, empowering people with knowledge they need to make the best decisions toward their natural good health. Rosemary encourages people to move the idea of prevention and natural health forward so that the people she works with can, in turn, help other people. She is a professional network marketer and wellness entrepreneur as well as founder and organizer for the Portland Natural Healing Group.

Rosemary is author of an upcoming book, *Loving Ginger,* and contributing author to other soon-to-be-published books on canine cancer and animal health. For more information, go to http://www.rosemaryssolutions.com.

Natalie Stemp and Simon

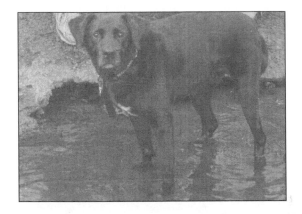

Owner's name: Natalie Stemp
Where they live: Washington D.C., Metro Area
Dog's name: Simon
Dog's breed: Labrador Retriever mix
Type of cancer: lymphoblastic lymphoma (a systemic cancer)
Age at diagnosis: 7 years
Prognosis: 1 month with no treatment; or an 80 percent chance at 6–9 months with chemotherapy
Outcome: 16 months and counting
Primary treatment: 19-week chemo protocol, cancer-fighting diet and supplement regimen, play time, massage (see blog for details)
Cancer Blog: http://www.simondogcancer.blogspot.com
Web address: http://www.calliopeboutique.com

Natalie Stemp is the proud owner of Simon, a Labrador Retriever who was diagnosed with lymphoma at the age of seven. As of November 2009, sixteen months after his initial diagnosis, Simon is back to his normal, silly self and is now deemed cancer-free.

Concerned by harmful production and wasteful consumerism, Natalie founded CalliopeBoutique, an online gift boutique with a unique philosophy: to help people "Live Exuberantly™." Knowing how important providing a chemical-free environment is to a dog fighting cancer, Calliope now offers cute, organic dog beds among many other goodies for people.

The company's mission is to leave a lighter footprint on the earth by helping people shop with a purpose and surround themselves and their loved ones with environmentally-friendly goods that inspire them, add something positive to their lives, and support artists and small business.

Karen Summers and Tensing

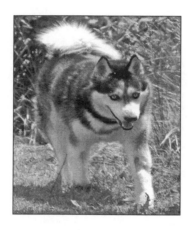

Owner's Name: Karen Summers
Where they live: Sparta, Missouri
Dog's name : Tensing
Dog's breed : Siberian Husky
Type of cancer : Lymphoma
Age at diagnosis : 7 years
Prognosis: 1 to 2 months without chemo and 12 to 18 months with chemo
Outcome: 2 years past original diagnosis
Primary treatment: University of Wisconsin, Madison chemo protocol, with prednisone
Email: justmekaren918@yahoo.com

Karen Summers had just lost her other dog Silver from Cushing's disease when Tensing, a rescue dog that had been kicked out of two homes, came into her life. It was love at first site. Tensing was a high-energy, ton-of-fun kind of dog. Playing was his life. Barely entering his senior years, Tensing was diagnosed with lymphoma. Using chemotherapy and prednisone, Karen was able to get two more quality years with her boy.

B Research Framework

Who: What is my dog's breed and what diseases is the breed predisposed to?

What: What is the type of cancer and how does it work?

Why: What possibly caused my dog's cancer?

> **NOTE:** This is not about blame, but about learning. For example, research shows that lawn pesticides are likely the cause of lymphoma. By knowing this, you can avoid its use as you move forward.

Where: Where are the tumors located?

When: How long does my veterinarian expect my dog to live?

How: How are others treating their dogs?

Example of a research map and the correlating action plan:

Who: Golden Retriever with no other Illnesses

Action plan: I found out that hemangiosarcoma is quite common in Golden Retrievers. I also learned what other diseases were prevalent in Goldens so I could ensure his treatment wouldn't possibly aggravate other possible risks.

What: Hemangiosarcoma

Action plan: Developed a custom treatment plan based on Cody's cancer. Cody's cancer caused bleeding tumors, so I had to be careful about blood thinning supplements. I also added a Chinese herb called Yunnan Paiyao to help with bleeding episodes.

Why: Genetics seems to play a big role in Cody's cancer. In addition, toxic substances (such as arsenic, vinyl chloride, and thorium dioxide) have been shown to cause this type of cancer in humans.

Action plan: I avoided all products with these toxins. For example, pressure treated wood used in the construction of decks, patios, and playgrounds prior to December 31, 2003, most likely contain arsenic, a proven carcinogen.

Where: Tumors in the heart, liver, and spleen

Action plan: In addition to implementing a regimen to fight the cancer overall, I added herbal support to help strengthen the affected organs: CoQ10 and hawthorn berry for his heart; milk thistle for his spleen; and a customized Chinese herbal blend from my holistic veterinarian for his spleen.

When: My veterinarians only gave Cody a few days to live.

Action plan: I found and communicated with dog owners fighting the same cancer that surpassed their prognosis. This helped me to stay positive.

How: Others are treating with surgery, chemo, and natural remedies

Action plan: I did so much reading that I started to see continual themes in treatment plans. It seemed there were a few dozen herbs and supplements used by most dog cancer survivors so I started with these.

C Dog Cancer Support Groups

Here is a partial list of online dog cancer support groups and a brief description of each.

Web Sites

- **FightDogCancer.com**—A social network that is also used as a support group; the site is committed to helping dog owners develop and manage their treatment plans based on previous dog cancer battles (custom built, designed especially for dog cancer). Users can earn points and donate them to dog cancer charities. http://www.fightdogcancer.com/

Yahoo! Groups

- **Artemisinin and Cancer**—This is a group for people who are using artemisinin and/or its analogs to treat their dogs' cancer or who are interested in networking with others who are using these experimental compounds. http://tinyurl.com/yl9zkjt [1]

- **Bone Cancer Dogs**—Dedicated to dogs with osteosarcoma and other bone cancers and to their guardians who fight bravely. It is a place for support, comfort, guidance, learning, encouragement and hope. http://tinyurl.com/yz73e55 [2]

---

1. pets.groups.yahoo.com/group/artemisinin_and_cancer/
2. pets.groups.yahoo.com/group/bonecancerdogs/

- **Canine Cancer**—Restricted to people whose dogs are currently battling cancer or are awaiting a definitive diagnosis. http://pets.groups.yahoo.com/group/CanineCancer/join

- **Canine Cancer Comfort**—Open to anyone who has or had a pet with cancer. http://pets.groups.yahoo.com/group/CanineCancerComfort/join

- **Pets with Cancer**—Open to anyone who has or had a pet (whether a dog, a cat, a horse) with cancer. http://pets.groups.yahoo.com/group/PetswithCancer/join

Nutrition Plans

Cody's Diet

Below is the basic recipe that I used for each meal. He was fed twice a day.

- 8 ounces organic meat (chicken, turkey, or beef)
- 2 teaspoons extra virgin olive oil
- 1–2 tablespoons fish oil
- 4 broccoli spears (slightly steamed and then finely chopped up)
- 1/2 can of sardines (in olive oil)
- 2 garlic cloves
- 1 teaspoon calcium carbonate (eggshells)

NOTE: Cody was a seventy-five-pound Golden Retriever, so you will want to adjust accordingly to your dog's weight, metabolism, and specific cancer. For example, high-protein diets are not recommended for dogs with kidney issues. Make sure you check with veterinarian.

Disnay's Diet

Disnay was fed three times per day, smaller amounts each feeding, consisting of grated bulk carrot, three raw cauliflower ears, and a grated broccoli stalk, which was divided into three portions for the daily feedings. The raw vegetables were mixed with bland chicken boiled in diluted chicken stock, just enough to flavor the vegetable mix.

Natural Flea and Tick Recipe

Cody's Natural Flea Spray

- 2 cups of lemon water (cut 3 lemons and boil in 2 cups of water; let steep overnight; then strain into a spray bottle)

- 5 drops of cedarwood oil (effective at repelling ticks and fleas)

- 5 drops of citronella oil

- 5 drops of peppermint oil

- 1 dropper full of rosemary extract

- 1 dropper full of vitamin E (acts as a natural preservative)

NOTE: I was fortunate enough to not live in a tick-infested area. I know they are tougher to deal with than fleas, but I have heard that rose geranium is another natural repellent. If I did live in such an area, I would add five drops of rose geranium to my flea formula and double the cedar to 10 drops.

Grief Counseling

- Association for Pet Loss and Bereavement:
  http://www.aplb.org/

- Lightening Strike Pet Loss Support Group:
  http://www.lightning-strike.com/

- Our Endlesslove Group Survivors and Angels:
  http://endlessloveangels.com

- Pet Loss Support Hotline:
  http://www.vet.cornell.edu/Org/Petloss/

- Pet Loss Support Page:
  http://www.pet-loss.net/index.shtml

- Petloss.com:
  http://www.petloss.com/

FightDogCancer.com

The online counterpart to *42 Rules to Fight Dog Cancer*, FightDogCancer.com is focused on gathering past and present dog cancer stories in one place so that those currently in battle can learn from our collective wisdom. Joining is free and users can earn points to raise funds for dog cancer charities.

The FightDogCancer.com service is built on three pillars: learn, act and support.

Learn: In order to fight dog cancer, you need to know what you are dealing with.

- Resource center complete with recommended books, links to dog cancer educational sites and online veterinarian ready to answer your questions immediately

- Social network so you can communicate with other dog owners fighting or who have fought dog cancer

Act: Once you arm yourself with knowledge, the next step is to determine your plan of action.

- Searchable database so you can see what other dog owners fighting the same battle have done and subsequent results

- Treatment plan spreadsheet to track and monitor changes or additions to your treatment plan

- Web site accessible to your entire dog cancer team online-from veterinarians to holistic practitioners—to ensure your entire team is communicating

Support: When fighting dog cancer, being supported and supporting others are critical to keeping you going.

- Blog feature so you create a tribute to your dog that will live on indefinitely so others will learn from your experience
- Group feature so you can start a focused group—whether for a specific type of cancer, breed or regional area
- Web site accessible to your friends and family to keep them updated on your dog cancer battle

FightDogCancer.com is not intended to replace the advice of a veterinary professional, and is for informational purposes only. Please seek the advice of your veterinarian or a veterinary specialist before giving your dog any supplements or pursuing any alternative cancer therapies.

References

i. Dr. William I. Lane and Linda Comac, *Sharks Don't Get Cancer: How Shark Cartilage Could Save Your Life* (Avery, 1992).

ii. University of Maryland Medical Center, "Hawthorn," http://tinyurl.com/yz8u5ym.[3]

iii. The Carcinogenic Potency Database, "Acrylamide: Rats and Mice: Cancer Test Summary," The Carcinogenic Potency Project, http://tinyurl.com/yzmo2yh.[4]

iv. U.S. Environmental Protection Agency, "Ground Water & Drinking Water FAQ," http://tinyurl.com/yl4jybs.[5]

v. Environmental Working Group, "A National Assessment of Tap Water Quality," 2005, http://tinyurl.com/yz9h7yx.[6]

vi. U.S. Environmental Protection Agency, "Indoor Air Quality: Residential Air Cleaners," http://www.epa.gov/iaq/pubs/residair.html.

---

3. www.umm.edu/altmed/articles/hawthorn-000256.htm
4. www.ncbi.nlm.nih.gov/pmc/articles/PMC1569423/pdf/envhper00452-0015.pdf
5. www.epa.gov/safewater/faq/faq.html
6. www.ewg.org/tap-water/executive-summary

vii. U.S. Environmental Protection Agency, Office of Research and Development, "The Total Exposure Assessment Methodology (TEAM) Study: Summary and Analysis Volume I," (June 1987), http://tinyurl.com/yz2m2nh.[7]

viii. U.S. Environmental Protection Agency, Office of Air and Radiation, "Report to Congress on Indoor Air Quality, Volume II: Assessment and Control of Indoor Air Pollution," 1989.

ix. Richard H. Pitcairn, DVM, PhD. *Dr. Pitcairn's Complete Guide to Natural Health for Dogs and Cats* (St. Martin's Press, 1995), 247.

x. Leigh Peterson, "Chemicals in Lawn Care Can Cause Cancer: Organic Lawn Care a Better Option for Your Pets and Family." Examiner.com, May 11, 2009, http://tinyurl.com/rxgljd.[8]

xi. Environmental Working Group, "Polluted Pets: High Levels of Toxic Industrial Chemicals Contaminate Cats and Dogs," April 17, 2008, http://www.ewg.org//book/export/html/26238.

xii. U.S. Environmental Protection Agency, Office of Air and Radiation, "Report to Congress on Indoor Air Quality, Volume II: Assessment and Control of Indoor Air Pollution," 1989.

xiii. U.S. Environmental Protection Agency, "An Introduction to Indoor Air Quality: Volatile Organic Compounds (VOCs)," http://www.epa.gov/iaq/voc.html.

xiv. Breast Cancer Fund, "Alkylphenols," http://tinyurl.com/38h3rdj.[9]

xv. WebVet, "Safe cleaning products for your pets," 2009, http://www.webvet.com/main/article?id=1355

xvi. Medical News Today, "AVMA: Advice To Owners Concerned About Lead In Toys," December 4, 2007, http://www.medicalnewstoday.com/articles/90653.php.

xvii. National Canine Foundation, 2010, http://www.wearethecure.org/.

xviii. Human Society, "U.S. Pet Ownership Statistics," 2010, http://tinyurl.com/ydhcrsa.[10]

---

7. oxposurescience.org/pub/reports/TEAM_Study_book_1987.pdf
8. www.examiner.com/x-10299-Cleveland-Pet-Products-Examiner~y2009m5d11-Chemicals-in-lawn-care-can-cause-cancer-organic-lawn-care-a-better-option-for-your-pets-and-family
9. www.breastcancerfund.org/clear-science/chemicals-glossary/alkylphenols.html
10. www.humanesociety.org/issues/pet_overpopulation/facts/pet_ownership_statistics.html

About the Author

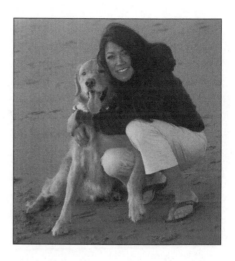

Aimee Quemuel is the author of *42 Rules to Fight Dog Cancer*. An avid animal advocate, having volunteered at the San Francisco SPCA, Pet's Unlimited, and the National Disaster Search Dog Foundation, Aimee is the "mamma" of two Golden Retrievers, beloved Cody and current dog CJ (shown in picture above), and founder of FightDogCancer.com, a site dedicated to helping dog owners fight dog cancer through the collective knowledge of dog owners throughout the world.

Aimee's journey began on November 5, 2006, when her beloved Cody collapsed after a day at the beach in San Francisco. He was rushed to the emergency veterinarian, where he was diagnosed with an incurable cancer, hemangiosarcoma. With tumors in his liver, spleen, and heart, Cody was given the grim prognosis of just a few weeks to live. Aimee was devastated, but could not let Cody go without a fight. After extensive research, her first step was to change his diet.

Unable to find freshly prepared, organic food critical to Cody's fight against cancer, Aimee started making Cody a "cancer-fighting" diet along with an arsenal of herbs and supplements. Cody thrived on his new diet and, long story short, survived seventeen months post his diagnosis to the age of twelve and a half years old. His veterinarians were amazed and coined him a miracle dog. Nearly two years after his death, Aimee decided to combine her life-changing experience with her career as a writer and marketing professional to write *42 Rules to Fight Dog Cancer.*

42 Rules Program

A lot of people would like to write a book, but only a few actually do. Finding a publisher, and distributing and marketing the book are challenges that prevent even the most ambitious authors from getting started.

If you want to be a successful author, we'll provide you the tools to help make it happen. Start today by completing a book proposal at our website **http://42rules.com/write/**.

For more information, email **info@superstarpress.com** or call 408-257-3000.

Other Happy About Books

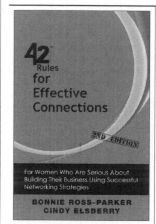

42 Rules™ for Effective Connections

For anyone who wants to improve communication, get better results in any networking environment and alleviate the stress and anxiety that comes from building a business where you have to go out to meet potential customers this book is a must-read.

Paperback: $19.95
eBook: $14.95

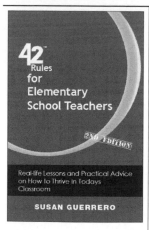

42 Rules™ for Elementary School Teachers

42 Rules for Elementary School Teachers is a collection of personal and practical professional advice on how to thrive as an elementary school teacher.

Paperback: $19.95
eBook: $14.95

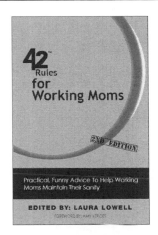

42 Rules™ for Working Moms

This book assembles the guidance of contributors who offer their thoughts on topics ranging from raising polite children and making time for yourself, as well as your mate, to losing the mommy guilt and delegating at home.

Paperback: $19.95
eBook: $14.95

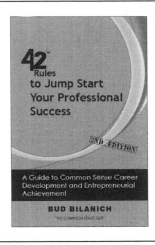

42 Rules™ to Jumpstart Your Professional Success

42 Rules to Jumpstart Your Personal and Professional Success is a guide to common sense career development, entrepreneurial achievement and life skills.

Paperback: $19.95
eBook: $14.95

Purchase these books at Happy About
http://happyabout.com
or at other online and physical bookstores.

A Message From Super Star Press™

Thank you for your purchase of this 42 Rules Series book. It is available online at:
http://www.happyabout.com/42rules/fightdogcancer.php or at other online and physical bookstores. To learn more about contributing to books in the 42 Rules series, check out **http://superstarpress.com**.

Please contact us for quantity discounts at **sales@superstarpress.com**.

If you want to be informed by email of upcoming books, please email **bookupdate@superstarpress.com**.

Made in the USA
San Bernardino, CA
10 January 2014